CYSTIC FIBROSIS

CYSTIC FIBROSIS

Edited by

DENNIS SHALE

David Davis Professor of Respiratory and Communicable Diseases,
University of Wales College of Medicine,
Llandough Hospital, Penarth

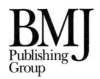

BMJ
Publishing
Group

© BMJ Publishing Group 1996

First published in 1996
by the BMJ Publishing Group, BMA House, Tavistock Square,
London WC1H 9JR

British Library Cataloguing in Publication Data

A catalogue record for this book is available from the British Library

ISBN 0-7279-0826-X

Typeset by Apek Typesetters Ltd, Nailsea, Bristol
Printed and bound in Great Britain by Latimer Trend Ltd, Plymouth

Contents

Preface

Cystic fibrosis was first described in children with fibrocystic disease of the pancreas. It comprised a syndrome of malabsorption and, if the child survived, chronic pulmonary infection. Since the late 1950s, median survival has increased from three to five years to between twenty five and thirty years, with a predicted median survival of forty years for children born in the present decade. These changes are due to many factors, chiefly the meticulous attention to nutrition and growth in childhood; the aggressive treatment of pulmonary infection; and the development of specialised centres for the management of both children and adults with cystic fibrosis.

A consequence of this is an increase in the total population with cystic fibrosis, particularly a growing proportion of adults. This increases the need for resources towards management of adult patients with chronic pulmonary infection and a range of extra conditions to those encountered in childhood, which include hepatic and biliary tract disease, diabetes mellitus, and problems of fertility. However, there remains a need for resources aimed at childhood with the continuing issues of prenatal and neonatal screening leading to possible prevention or earlier diagnosis. A separate and as yet poorly perceived issue is population screening, which may have an impact on total patient numbers in years to come.

This book aims to present both current clinical thinking and practice with more fundamental aspects relating to the pathophysiology of cystic fibrosis. To do this an international based group of scientists and clinicians with interests in cystic fibrosis has been asked to provide commentaries on relevant areas. In addition to the clinical advances, there has been an enormous development in our understanding in terms of the genetics and molecular biology of cystic fibrosis. Currently cystic fibrosis is at the "cutting edge" of scientific endeavour in respect of the understanding of the biology of genetic diseases; the potential for gene transfer and therapy; and the application of sophisticated molecular biology and protein biochemistry methodologies to clinical medicine. I hope that this book achieves some of its aims in covering such a diverse and rapidly expanding field.

In all areas of clinical and scientific activity there is debate, controversy, and, occasionally, frank disagreement. In the following chapters some of these are reviewed as they often represent gaps in knowledge and act as a spur to further research and development. In cystic fibrosis it is the next decade that holds so much promise and excitement to us as scientists and clinicians, but above all for our patients, for whom there is the promise of a potential cure for some aspects of the disease and a normal life span. These enormous changes in cystic fibrosis are due to the close liaison between science and medicine, giving a model for the future elucidation and management of complex disorders.

Dennis Shale
November 1995

1 Management in children

E JOAN HILLER

The diagnosis of cystic fibrosis comes as a shock to most parents, and it may take some time before they accept it and learn about the disease and its management. It is essential for members of the cystic fibrosis team to spend as much time as necessary in the early months with the family, not only to educate them about the condition and practical aspects of management, but also to help them work through their emotional reactions. This will pay dividends later, as the successful management of cystic fibrosis in childhood is impossible without the full involvement of well motivated parents. It is the daily care that the child gets at home that is really important, and this is demanding and time consuming.

Until effective gene treatment becomes a reality there is no cure. Supportive treatment, however, is both available and worthwhile with the aims of preventing or delaying lung damage; maintaining good nutrition; preventing complications, or at least diagnosing and treating them early; and enabling the child and family to live as normal a life as possible. This requires regular supervision, careful attention to detail, and continuing family education and support.

The lungs

Prevention of respiratory infection should be attempted where possible. Parents should be advised not to smoke in the home or to take the baby into smoky places. Babies with cystic fibrosis should avoid contact with older children and adults with respiratory infections. They should be fully immunised, particularly against pertussis and measles, and influenza vaccination should be recommended each autumn.

Treatment

The aims are to keep the airways clear of excessive secretions and to treat intercurrent infection effectively.[1]

Physiotherapy

Parents should be taught techniques of postural drainage appropriate to the age of the child and advised to treat the child at least twice daily and more often if the cough increases. While it is difficult to prove the value of such treatment in infancy, it is well accepted then and we hope will become part of the daily routine throughout life. As the child grows older, physiotherapy techniques should be reviewed regularly by a physiotherapist experienced in the care of cystic fibrosis and an appropriate wedge or tipping frame provided. Children can be introduced to the active cycle of breathing and "huffing" quite early, and the use of a positive expiratory pressure (PEP) mask may enable them to undertake at least part of their own treatment.

Exercise

Regular exercise should be encouraged from an early age. Small trampolines are excellent for preschool children. Many parents will restrict their children's participation in sport at school and this should be countered with an explanation of the benefits of such activities. Teenagers should keep up some sort of exercise but are often reluctant to do so.

Antibiotic treatment

Antibiotic treatment should usually be based on the results of cultures of sputum or cough swabs, which should be taken regularly.[2] Most acute infections in young children are caused by viruses for which no specific treatment is available, though ribavirin should be considered for bronchiolitis caused by respiratory syncitial virus. There is evidence that viral infections allow bacteria to colonise the respiratory tract,[3] so it is usual to treat all exacerbations of symptoms. In the absence of positive cultures it is wise to cover both *Staphylococcus aureus* and *Haemophilus influenzae* (Table 1.1). Antibiotics should be given orally in high dosage for a minimum of 10–14 days, as the response may be slow.

Staph aureus is an important pathogen in children with cystic fibrosis, though it is less common than in the past. Some clinics advise regular "prophylactic" flucloxacillin for varying periods of

Table 1.1 Antibiotic treatment

Pathogen	Drug	Dose (mg/kg/day)	Route	Duration (days)
H influenzae	Amoxycillin	50–100	Orally	10–14
	Co-amoxiclav	50–100	Orally	10–14
	Co-trimoxazole	96	Orally	10–14
Staph aureus	Flucloxacillin	100	Orally	28 or more
	Erythromycin	50	Orally	28 or more
	Sodium fusidate	50	Orally	28 or more
	Clindamycin	20–30	Orally	28 or more
	Vancomycin	40	Intravenously	10–14
Ps aeruginosa	Ciprofloxacin	15–30	Orally	14–21
	Azlocillin	300	Intravenously	14
	Ceftazidime	150	Intravenously	14
	Tobramycin	9–10	Intravenously	14
	Gentamicin	Adjust according to blood concentration		
	Aztreonam	150–200	Intravenously	14
	Imipenem	30–90	Intravenously	14
	Colomycin*		Nebulised	

*0.5–2 MU twice daily

time, though there is little evidence of benefit and the organism may still be isolated from the sputum. The alternative is to culture the sputum regularly and treat Staph aureus when it is isolated, irrespective of symptoms, to try to eradicate it. This may be difficult, and require repeated and prolonged courses of antibiotics.

Although strains of H influenzae may be normal commensals of the upper respiratory tract, isolates from children with cystic fibrosis may be associated with increased symptoms and should be treated.[4]

Once infection with Pseudomonas species becomes established it is impossible to eradicate for any length of time, but appropriate antibiotic treatment improves lung function and symptoms with a reduction in the inflammatory response.[5] The beneficial response to treatment tends to decrease as the lung disease progresses. Ciprofloxacin is the only antibiotic available with activity against Pseudomonas that can be taken orally and it is widely used although not licensed for use in childhood because of problems with the joints in young animals. Arthropathy has proved to be uncommon in practice and has been reversed when the drug was stopped. Photosensitive skin rashes are more common. Unfortunately, pseudomonads quickly become resistant to ciprofloxacin, so it is unsuitable for frequent or prolonged use. Treatment with intravenous antibiotics is often required and is usually well tolerated though allergic skin rashes may occur. The antibiotics given are chosen on the basis of recent bacterial sensitivities, previous responses, and known allergies. Multiple resistance is an increasing problem, though the clinical response does not always parallel the *in vitro* sensitivity pattern. The use of neonatal long lines or implanted devices such as the Port-a-Cath, and the liberal use of lignocaine and prilocaine (Emla) cream makes intravenous antibiotic treatment less traumatic for the child.

With appropriate training and supervision, many parents can give intravenous antibiotic treatment successfully at home and this is much preferred by many families.[6] The introduction of the Homecare system, which delivers ready prepared individual doses to the home in the elastomeric Intermate giving set, has helped by reducing the time needed to prepare each dose and removing the need for an infusion pump. It is expensive but cost-effective

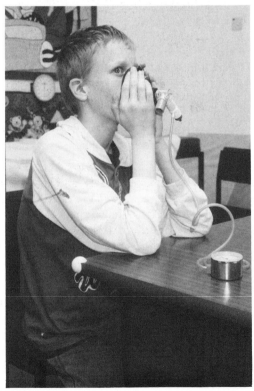

Boy using PEP mask. (Reproduced with parents' permission)

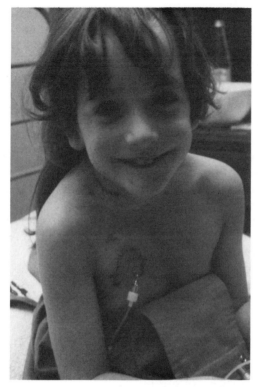

Girl with Port-a-Cath in her chest wall. (Reproduced with parents' permission)

because it reduces the number of hospital admissions. Home intravenous treatment still causes anxiety, and appropriate nursing support is needed as well as easy access to the ward if the line needs replacing or the child's condition deteriorates.

Intravenous antibiotic treatment is demanding, time consuming, and expensive, and is usually given when the patient's symptoms warrant it, supported by a deterioration in lung function or loss of

---

Organisms that are important in children with cystic fibrosis

- *Staph aureus*
- *H influenzae*
- *Ps aeruginosa*
- *B cepacia*

---

weight, or both. Some clinics follow the Copenhagen practice of giving regular three monthly courses of treatment. There is no evidence from prospective controlled trials to support this practice, and the results of the British Thoracic Society multicentre study currently in progress are awaited with interest.

Nebulised antibiotic treatment, usually with gentamicin, tobramycin, or colomycin benefits patients with moderate or severe lung disease.[7] It is given either in the short or the long term, twice daily after physiotherapy using a mouth tube, appropriate nebuliser unit and a powerful compressor. Compliance with this rather tedious form of treatment is often poor, but may be improved by negotiating a period off treatment in the summer in exchange for cooperation during the winter.

Nebulised colomycin in combination with oral ciprofloxacin delays the establishment of chronic pseudomonal colonisation when given for three weeks after the first isolation of the organism and repeated when it is re-isolated until it is well established.[8] This seems a useful approach and, because it does not require hospital admission, has been well accepted.

Bronchodilators

Many children with cystic fibrosis have some degree of reversible airflow obstruction, which often varies in severity. Their response to bronchodilator treatment should be tested with peak flow measurements at intervals and, if there is a useful improvement, regular β-agonist treatment should be given before physiotherapy. This may also be needed to prevent the airflow obstruction which may result from inhaling nebulised colistin. Some children have asthma in addition to cystic fibrosis and will benefit from regular preventive treatment.

Mucolytics

Oral cough medicines or mucolytics are rarely helpful, but the inhalation of nebulised n-acetylcysteine (Parvolex) may help expectoration in patients with thick sputum. It should be diluted at least 50:50 with saline, and not used if it results in haemoptyses. DNase is more effective, though the recommended groups of patients so far studied have had mild lung disease.

Corticosteroids

Oral prednisolone is indicated if there is good evidence of allergic bronchopulmonary aspergillosis, or if the patient has acute asthma. Wheezing is common in young children with cystic fibrosis and the response to corticosteroids is often disappointing. Although such treatment may improve general wellbeing, there is little overall evidence of benefit in most patients. Side effects, particularly diabetes, are common.

Oxygen

Hypoxaemia, particularly at night, is common in advanced lung disease and patients often benefit from oxygen. Few children will tolerate this for more than short periods during the day, but feel better and are more active if they use it intermittently and particularly during sleep. An oxygen concentrator at home is needed, with a low flow meter and a nasal cannula.

Lung transplantation

Successful transplants have been undertaken in childhood after appropriate assessment, but there are many problems and a great shortage of donors.[9]

Terminal care

The rate of deterioration is variable, as is the determination of individual children and families to keep fighting. Most parents recognise when the end is in sight for their child and wish it to be peaceful. It is important to recognise this and to discuss with the family the need to accept the situation and to adjust treatment to provide effective control of distressing symptoms, as far as possible. A community paediatric nursing service allows most patients to die at home if they wish, with appropriate support. An intravenous infusion of morphine or diamorphine is the most effective way of relieving breathlessness and anxiety in the last days, the dose being adjusted as necessary. If in hospital privacy and quiet should be ensured, aggressive treatment discontinued, and cardiopulmonary resuscitation or ventilation not attempted.

Nutrition

Many children are underweight at the time of diagnosis, and poor growth in later years is a common problem. This is not only the result of pancreatic insufficiency, but also inadequate intake associated with chronic lung disease, and a raised resting energy expenditure.[10] Better nourished patients seem to survive longer,[11]

> Better nourished children survive longer, so growth should be monitored regularly and diet supervised by an experienced dietitian

so children's growth should be monitored regularly and their management supervised by an experienced dietitian.

Most patients with cystic fibrosis require enzyme supplements throughout life, using one of the enteric-coated microsphere preparations now available. For babies, the capsule is opened and the microspheres given from a spoon with a little fluid. It is important to emphasise that the child must not chew the microspheres and that they must be given with every meal or snack. Ideally, the dose should be titrated to faecal fat measurements, but these are not available in most hospitals. Stool weights are a useful alternative if the family can be persuaded to cooperate. Otherwise, the dose is adjusted to achieve stools that are as normal as possible and the child gaining weight satisfactorily.

Some children take large doses of pancreatic enzymes and may benefit from the use of an H_2 blocker such as cimetidine to block gastric acid secretion as a low pH in the upper small bowel (caused by lack of pancreatic bicarbonate secretion) reduces enzyme activity. More recently omeprazole has been used in some patients with benefit. Recently the use of high lipase concentration enzyme replacement has become popular with both patients and professionals, but the reported link with colitis, colonic strictures, and the need for major abdominal surgery has led to such products no longer being recommended in children.[12] The Committee of Safety of Medicines has also advised that the total daily dose of lipase should not exceed 10 000 units/kg/day of any pancreatic enzyme preparation.

Diet

Good eating habits must be established early and the family educated about how to provide a high calorie, nutritionally satisfactory diet. Mixed feeding often has to be started early, but otherwise babies do not usually need any special measures to ensure good weight gain. Parents may be restricting the family's fat intake to prevent heart disease and find it strange to be advised to give the child with cystic fibrosis a high fat intake, but this is necessary to ensure that adequate calories are given and is well tolerated provided that adequate enzymes are also taken.

Most children grow satisfactorily until adolescence provided that they have an adequate intake and appropriate pancreatic enzyme supplements. High calorie supplementary feeds are needed only during or after periods of illness and should not be given routinely. They are, however, useful for children who are unable to achieve an adequate calorie intake and weight gain because of anorexia or excessive fussiness.

It may be extremely difficult to maintain an adequate intake in some children, particularly adolescents with severe lung disease. These patients may benefit considerably from overnight nasogastric tube feeding or gastrostomy feeding for short or long periods; this gives improved weight gain and self-image though rarely causes any real improvement in lung function.

Vitamins

Malabsorption of fat-soluble vitamins is common and supplements should be given. Adequate doses of vitamins A, D and E should be given to maintain normal blood concentrations. Non-compliance is common and blood concentrations should be checked regularly. Recommended doses vary considerably (Table 1.2). There is no suitable multivitamin preparation which includes vitamin E at present, so this must be given separately. Vitamin deficiencies are uncommon, but there is some evidence that low concentrations of vitamin A develop more often in patients with more severe disease, particularly if the liver is involved.[13]

Other gastrointestinal problems

Continued gastrointestinal symptoms and poor growth, despite individualised management as described, require further investigation. Gastro-oesophageal reflux is common in patients with cystic fibrosis, and both coeliac disease and Crohn's disease have been described in such patients.

Table 1.2 Recommended vitamin supplements

Vitamin	Dose/day
A	3000–8000 IU
D	400–800 IU
E	50–200 mg

Meconium ileus

Up to 20% of infants with cystic fibrosis present with neonatal bowel obstruction. At least one third of these infants can be treated satisfactorily with a contrast enema examination, which must be undertaken by an experienced paediatric radiologist and a paediatric surgeon. Operation will be required if this fails, or if there is perforation of the bowel. Postoperatively there may be some delay before the bowel functions, and total parenteral nutrition may be required. Temporary food intolerances are common, and a special feed may be required for a few weeks.

Distal intestinal obstruction syndrome (meconium ileus equivalent)

Faecal retention causes abdominal pain and a palpable mass in the right iliac fossa. Early treatment with oral lactulose and n-acetylcysteine (Fabrol) may resolve the problem; if not, it can be followed by oral sodium and methyl glucamine diatrizoates (Gastrografin) which is usually effective.[14] If there is subacute obstruction the choice of treatment lies between a contrast enema examination, given under radiological control, and the use of an oral lavage solution.[15]

Liver disease

Although about 10% of patients with cystic fibrosis have abnormal liver function tests, symptoms of hepatocellular failure are uncommon. Portal hypertension develops in a proportion, but may be extremely slow to progress. Bleeding from oesophageal varices requires endoscopy and sclerotherapy, but such treatment is not recommended before bleeding occurs.

The use of ursodeoxycholic acid improves liver function tests in the short term, but it is not yet known whether it will prevent or delay the development of cirrhosis and portal hypertension.[16]

Electrolyte disturbances

Salt depletion (heat stroke) may occur in hot weather or if the child is febrile, and requires salt tablets or extra salt in the diet as well as additional fluids. A metabolic alkalosis (pseudo-Bartter's syndrome) sometimes develops in infants and should be suspected if there is severe failure to thrive despite adequate intake and enzyme therapy; potassium or sodium chloride supplements, or both, are needed.[17]

Diabetes

There is an increasing incidence of diabetes mellitus with increasing age. It is unusual in young children, but tends to present with loss of weight in teenagers. Ketoacidosis is rare, but temporary glucose intolerance related to infection or corticosteroid treatment is quite common. Insulin treatment is needed and the diabetes is usually stable and easy to control. It is important to continue the high calorie diet for cystic fibrosis and not to allow a standard diabetic diet to be imposed.

Continuing supervision and care

Patients with cystic fibrosis need regular hospital supervision throughout life. Continuity of experienced medical care is important, which means that the consultant must see the family regularly, if possible in a special cystic fibrosis clinic with adequate time for proper review and discussion. Height, weight, and lung function should be measured every two or three months and the child examined. A sputum specimen or cough swab should always be sent for culture.

Experienced dietetic, physiotherapy, and nursing staff are essential, both in the clinic and on the ward. Such a multi-disciplinary team is likely to be found only in a clinic that treats a large number of patients with cystic fibrosis and, ideally, all such patients should attend a specialist centre, or have some form of shared care arrangement.[18] An annual review of the child's condition with a chest radiograph, measurement of liver function tests and vitamin concentrations, and other investigations if relevant, combined with a physiotherapist's and dietitian's review, is helpful to assess progress and review management.

Recent problems with *Burkholderia cepacia* have led to recommendations that clinics should segregate patients with this pathogen from others and that these patients should be nursed in isolation, which creates both practical and social problems.

A chronic illness like cystic fibrosis, with an uncertain prognosis, puts a great strain on families. Continued skilled social work is essential, but often difficult to obtain. Help may be needed with housing, travel, finances, obtaining appropriate allowances, and

11

bereavement, as well as general practical and emotional support to enable the family to provide the care required.

Genetic counselling

All parents need to know at an early stage that there is a one in four risk of another sibling being affected and most will welcome referral to a genetic clinic for discussion of antenatal diagnosis if another pregnancy is planned. Detection of carriers should be offered to relatives and their partners where appropriate.

As children with cystic fibrosis grow older the team may need to liaise with schools and community services to provide appropriate information and extra help for the patients. Teenagers need help to become as independent as possible, particularly with physiotherapy. Appropriate career guidance should be given early. Transfer to an adult cystic fibrosis clinic can be quite difficult, but should be planned in advance and eased with visits or joint clinics so that the change is made when the patient is ready.

References

1 Hodson ME, Warner JO. Respiratory problems and their treatment. *Br Med Bull* 1992; **48**: 931–48.
2 Hiller EJ. The rational use of antibiotics in cystic fibrosis. *Paediatric Respiratory Medicine* 1993; **1**: 20–3.
3 Peterson NT, Høiby N, Mordhorst CH, Lund K, Flensborg EW, Bruun B. Respiratory infections in cystic fibrosis caused by virus, chlamydia and mycoplasma – possible synergism with Ps. aeruginosa. *Acta Paediatr Scand* 1981; **70**: 623–8.
4 Rayner RJ, Hiller EJ, Ispahani P, Baker M. Haemophilus infection in cystic fibrosis. *Arch Dis Child* 1990; **65**: 255–8.
5 Høiby N. Pseudomonas infection in cystic fibrosis. In: Dodge JA, Brock DJH, Widdicombe JH, eds. *Cystic fibrosis: current topics.* Chichester: John Wiley, 1993; 251–68.
6 David TJ. Intravenous antibiotics at home in children with cystic fibrosis. *J R Soc Med* 1989; **82**: 130–1.
7 Littlewood JM, Smye SW, Cunliffe H. Aerosol antibiotic treatment in cystic fibrosis. *Arch Dis Child* 1993; **68**: 788–92.
8 Valerius NH, Koch C, Høiby N. Prevention of chronic Pseudomonas aeruginosa colonisation in cystic fibrosis by early treatment. *Lancet* 1991; **338**: 725–6.
9 Warner J. Heart lung transplantation: all the facts. *Arch Dis Child* 1991; **66**: 1013–17.
10 Durie PR, Pencharz PB. A rational approach to the nutritional care of patients with cystic fibrosis. *J R Soc Med* 1989; **82**: 11–20.
11 Corey M, McLaughlin FJ, Williams M, Levison H. A comparison of survival, growth and pulmonary function in patients with cystic fibrosis in Boston and Toronto. *J Clin Epidemiol* 1988; **41**: 583–91.
12 Smyth RL, van Velzen D, Smyth AR, Lloyd DA, Heaf DP. Strictures of

ascending colon in cystic fibrosis and high strength pancreatic enzymes. *Lancet* 1994; **343**: 85–6.

13 Rayner RJ. Fat soluble vitamins in cystic fibrosis. *Proc Nutr Soc* 1992; **51**: 245–50.

14 O'Halloran SM, Gilbert J, McKendrick DM, Carty HMC, Heaf D. Gastrografin in acute meconium ileus equivalent. *Arch Dis Child* 1986; **61**: 1128–30.

15 Cleghorn GJ, Forstner GG, Stringer DA, Durie PR. Treatment of distal intestinal obstruction syndrome in cystic fibrosis with a balanced intestinal lavage solution. *Lancet* 1986; **i**: 8–11.

16 Williams SGJ, Westaby D, Tanner MS, Mowat A. Liver and biliary problems in cystic fibrosis. *Br Med Bull* 1992; **48**: 877–92.

17 Devlin J, Beckett NS, David TJ. Elevated sweat potassium, hyperaldosteronism and pseudo-Bartter's syndrome: a spectrum of disorders associated with cystic fibrosis. *J R Soc Med* 1989; **82**: 38–43.

18 David TJ. The case for cystic fibrosis centres. *J R Soc Med* 1987; **80**: 51–4.

2 Management in adults

DENNIS SHALE

Much of the care of adults is similar to that of children and involves chiefly maintenance of body weight, nutrition, and lung function. There do, however, remain issues that are peculiar to adults, such as male fertility, pregnancy, meconium ileus equivalent, and the development of diabetes mellitus or liver disease. Additional to clinical problems is the burden of social and psychological adaptations to adult life and the prospect of limited survival (see Chapter 9).

The main preoccupation of the physician caring for adults with cystic fibrosis is the respiratory system, failure of which is the principal cause of death, though comprehensive care of this multisystem disorder is essential. This chapter will concentrate mainly on lung disease.

Clinical features of lung disease

The major respiratory symptoms are dyspnoea, the chronic production of purulent sputum with occasional haemoptysis, tightness of the chest with occasional wheeze, and reduced exercise tolerance. The severity of these symptoms varies with the extent of destruction of the lung, and acutely with events such as viral infection.

Examination may show combinations of the following signs depending on the severity of the lung disease: cyanosis, clubbing, dyspnoea, abnormal chest shape (for example, pectus carinatum), intercostal indrawing, overinflation of the thorax, wheezing, and scattered coarse crackles throughout the lung fields. Exacerbations of such symptoms are often associated with weight loss and underline the characteristic unpredictability of the progression of pulmonary disease in cystic fibrosis.

Investigations

The diagnosis of cystic fibrosis is usually made in childhood, though some patients remain undiagnosed until their second or third decade. In such patients gastrointestinal and pulmonary involvement may be mild, so that cystic fibrosis is not considered.[1] Diagnosis, as in children, is based on symptoms, signs, and a positive sweat test, although the latter must be carefully interpreted as sweat electrolyte concentrations tend to be greater in adults.[2] Diagnosis is usually confirmed by ascertaining the patient's genotype.

In most adults investigations are related to monitoring progression of pulmonary disease or the involvement of other organ systems. Most centres carry out an annual review, though the extent of such reviews varies.

Radiology

Most adult patients have abnormal chest radiographs. Overinflation can usually be detected in adults, and thickening of the bronchial wall appears as circular lesions or tram lines on the radiograph; bronchiectasis is seen as cysts and rounded opacities which progress to larger lesions. Fibrosis also develops causing increased background shadowing, and blebs or small bullae (a potential cause of pneumothorax) may be seen apically.

Conventional chest radiography is the main method of monitoring lung disease in adults, and is essential to assess complications such as pneumothorax, haemoptysis, abscess formation, segmental or lobar opacification, pulmonary hypertension, and cor pulmonale.

Annual assessment

Every year:
  Full examination and history
  Comprehensive assessment of respiratory function, including reversibility of airflow limitation by bronchodilator treatment
  Oxygen saturation at rest and following exercise
  Chest radiograph (posterior-anterior and lateral)
  Blood concentrations of vitamins A, E and D and inflammatory markers
When clinically indicated:
  Ultrasound assessment of the liver and gastrointestinal system
  Full dietary assessment over a four day period

15

Scoring systems based on an assessment of hyperinflation and linear and nodular opacities have been devised, usually for children, and can be used to monitor progression, though they are less sensitive in adults.[3, 4] Many centres use the Chrispin-Norman, Brasfield, or Northern scoring systems in the annual assessment of patients.[3-5] In the upper airways there is often poor development and opacification of the facial sinus.

High resolution computed tomography usually enhances changes detected in the plain radiograph, and additionally shows the distribution of bronchiectasis.[6 7] Evidence of lung involvement can be seen in the scan when the chest radiograph may still look normal, giving earlier information on lung disease. The changes detected by scanning relate more to known lung disease, such as mucus plugging, consolidation, and bronchiectasis, than features in the chest radiograph. Scoring systems based on specific changes have been developed but are not used routinely.[7]

Pulmonary function tests

Spirometry and peak expiratory flow rate (PEFR) are used to monitor progression of airways disease and response to treatment. Most centres record these at each visit as trends help to plan management interventions such as transplantation. The tests usually show an obstructive pattern, with reduced forced expiratory volume in one second (FEV_1) and PEFR. More sophisticated measurements may indicate overinflation with an increased total lung capacity and residual volume.

Exercise testing is a sensitive indicator of pulmonary impairment with a reduction in exercise tolerance as destruction of the lungs progresses.

Arterial blood gas tensions and oxygen saturation

Progressive destruction of the lungs leads to respiratory failure. Type I failure can be diagnosed from arterial blood gas measurements or arterialised ear lobe capillary blood. Transcutaneous oxygen saturation is a non-invasive alternative that is often used at routine clinic visits but it is not sensitive to mild hypoxaemia.

In type II failure oximetry is less useful as knowledge of $PaCO_2$, pH, and bicarbonate concentration is also needed to assess progression or resolution of this problem. Symptoms such as morning headaches or tremor may indicate the need to measure $PaCO_2$. Assessment of saturation is useful for monitoring supplementary oxygen treatment, provided that carbon dioxide retention has been ruled out.

Management of pulmonary infections

Patients should avoid people known to have respiratory infections such as the common cold. Annual immunisation against influenza should be recommended, particularly if an epidemic is expected. For bacterial infections antibiotics may be given orally, by aerosol, or intravenously, as in childhood.

Staphylococcus aureus

Staph aureus remains a pathogen in many adults. In most centres adults are treated whenever *Staph aureus* is isolated, often with the aim of eradication. This may require prolonged treatment, usually with flucloxacillin or erythromycin if the patient is symptom free and with the addition of either fusidic acid or clindamycin if symptoms develop (see Table 1.1).

Haemophilus influenzae

Total or partial eradication of *H influenzae* is also possible. Treatment is usually with ampicillin or amoxycillin or an amoxycillin-clavulanic acid combination. The use of ampicillin or amoxycillin may be limited by the presence of β-lactamase producing strains, and if so tetracycline, cephalosporins, erythromycin, clarithromycin, ciprofloxacin, ofloxacin, or chloramphenicol are possible effective options (see Table 1.1).

Pseudomonas aeruginosa

Prevention of acquisition and colonisation
Over 80% of adult patients are chronically infected with *Ps aeruginosa*, often in combination with other bacteria, though for those that are not colonised attempts at prevention are worthwhile. Allocation to specific clinic sessions or wards based on the presence or absence of *Ps aeruginosa* or antibiotic resistance patterns reduces the rate of acquisition and the risk of the spread of multiresistant organisms,[8] though nosocomial spread is unusual.[9] Eradication is not usually possible once colonisation is established,[9] but vigorous treatment with nebulised colomycin and oral ciprofloxacin for

17

three weeks at the first isolation and for longer periods at subsequent isolations may delay colonisation (see Table 1.1).[10]

Management of chronic infection

The options are to treat clinically defined exacerbations; to treat electively irrespective of symptoms for two weeks at three monthly intervals; or a combination of these regimens.[11] Antibiotics are usually given intravenously for progressive worsening of respiratory symptoms, though usually the cause of an exacerbation is unknown. Various definitions of an exacerbation are used, though an increase in volume or purulence of sputum; a reduction in baseline respiratory function (for example, FEV_1 or PEFR reduced by more than 10% of best recorded value in the last 12 months); weight loss; lethargy; and breathlessness can all be taken as indicators for antibiotic treatment, because fever and leucocytosis are not particularly common.[12]

Giving treatment only at the time of exacerbation has the disadvantage that lung injury is continuous with evidence of inflammatory activity returning to pretreatment levels between episodes of clinical deterioration.[12, 13] Intermittent elective treatment has the disadvantage of occupying up to eight weeks each year and in Copenhagen when they initially adopted this policy, there was concern about the development of multiresistant infections. A combination of this approach, with a policy of segregation reduced the risk.[11] There has been no controlled trial of this pattern of antibiotic treatment though good survival results have been reported from Copenhagen and from other centres that adopted the policy.[11]

Most centres treat with two antibiotics given intravenously for 10–14 days whether their policy is elective or on demand (see Table 1.1). Improvement in lung function and the maximum reduction in the bacterial count in the sputum occur between 7–10 days.[14] Treatment may be given in hospital or at home. For frequent treatment an implanted device in the chest wall or antecubital fossa such as a Port-a-Cath or Pas-Port, solves the problems of venous access. Fine bore paediatric lines help to preserve peripheral veins and are acceptable to patients who need less frequent courses of antibiotic treatment.

Most antibiotic regimens include a carboxypenicillin (carbenicillin or ticarcillin) or ureidopenicillin (azlocillin or piperacillin), and an aminoglycoside (tobramycin, gentamicin, netilmicin or amikacin) (see Table 1.1). Ceftazidime or cefsulodin may be used instead of penicillin. Ceftazidime is an effective single agent making it highly acceptable for intravenous treatment at home.[12] Other choices include aztreonam and colistin, though the latter is most widely used in an aerosol. Doses tend to be larger than normal in patients with cystic fibrosis because of their more rapid clearance of antibiotics. Clinical studies suggest little difference between these combinations in regard to patient benefit measured in clinical or inflammatory terms,[12] and the role of antibiotics in the treatment of clinical exacerbations has been questioned.

Oral treatment with a quinolone such as ciprofloxacin or ofloxacin is an alternative, and may avoid a course of intravenous treatment. Oral treatment is often limited by the rapid acquisition of *in vitro* resistance, though the importance of this is unclear as sensitivity testing is of limited value in patients with chronic colonisation.[15]

Continuous treatment for chronic infection

The benefit of continuous antibiotic treatment given orally has not been confirmed and resistance to the antibiotic is likely to develop. Nebulised antibiotics (initially carbenicillin and later gentamicin, tobramycin and colistin) are beneficial and safe when used long term. Colistin and tobramycin in particular provide benefit and preserve lung function when used over long periods.[16,17]

Burkholderia cepacia (formerly Pseudomonas cepacia)

This organism is a motile Gram negative rod that causes onion rot, but is not usually pathogenic in man. In cystic fibrosis it is a nosocomial pulmonary pathogen, though its prevalence is only 3%–6% in adult patients.[18-20]

Because of its potential for nosocomial spread colonised patients are usually separated from non-colonised patients.[20-22] Segregation in hospital alone will not reduce the acquisition rate of *B cepacia* because of social contact between patients. Various national associations have produced guidelines for patients, their families, and the medical profession, on the rationale for separation.[23,24] Generally, they advise that *B cepacia* is most likely to be caught through close contact with a colonised person. To be effective a separation policy requires that the culture of *B cepacia* is effective and equally good in all centres, so that infected patients are identified and do not remain in contact with uninfected patients.

This may not be so and microbiological services must ensure standardised procedures for the culture of *B cepacia*.

Recommendations include: colonised and uninfected patients should have separate clinic and inpatient facilities, and there should be better hygiene among medical staff, including hand-washing after seeing each patient. Separation is also recommended at social gatherings outside the hospital.

The Cystic Fibrosis Trust of Great Britain recommended that:[24] patients known to carry *B cepacia* should not attend organised meetings, conferences, or group events at which uninfected people are likely to be present, and that carriers of *B cepacia* should ensure that non-colonised people do not attend special events organised for patients colonised with *B cepacia* and that those colonised with *B cepacia* should avoid close contact with young children with cystic fibrosis.

The Cystic Fibrosis Foundation in the United States has banned holiday camps for patients because of the risk of transmission of *B cepacia*. The British Cystic Fibrosis Trust defined low, medium, and high risk activities. Low risk activities are defined as casual meetings indoors or outdoors such as branch meetings; medium risk as handshaking, sharing rooms at conferences, and social kissing; and high risk as sharing eating or drinking utensils and intimate contact. An effective segregation policy requires well informed patients, and health professionals who are willing to provide support for the emotional, psychological, and social impact of this infection on patients their friends and their families.

There are three distinct clinical patterns of *B cepacia* infection:
- Chronic asymptomatic carriage, sometimes in combination with *Ps aeruginosa*
- Progressive deterioration over many months with recurrent fever, weight loss, and repeated hospital admissions similar to end stage *Ps aeruginosa* infection
- A rapidly progressive and usually fatal deterioration in patients who may previously have been considered to be only mildly affected.[22-28]

The choice of antibiotic for the treatment of *B cepacia* is often confounded by the development of resistance and the organism is initially likely to be more resistant to antibiotics than *Ps aeruginosa*. Eradication is unlikely and effective antibiotic treatment is confined largely to ceftazidime, tobramycin, co-trimoxazole, or chloramphenicol, which reinforces the need to prevent spread between patients.

Other infections

Allergic bronchopulmonary aspergillosis affects up to 15% of patients, and its diagnosis and treatment are identical to those when it is associated with other respiratory conditions. Mycobacterial infections including atypical organisms are being increasingly diagnosed in patients with cystic fibrosis. Such infections should be sought in patients who continue to deteriorate despite appropriate antibiotic treatment of other known infections. Treatment of tuberculosis or atypical mycobacterial infection is identical to that in patients who do not have cystic fibrosis.

Physiotherapy

As in children, physiotherapy is a major part of the treatment of adults with chronic respiratory infection. Various methods, including postural drainage, accompanied by percussion, deep breathing, and directed coughing with forced expiratory manoeuvres are used to increase expectoration. Some patients prefer a positive expiratory pressure mask which may improve their compliance.

Regular exercise is a popular option for young adults. It improves cardiopulmonary fitness and the sense of wellbeing, but there is no evidence that it improves expectoration of sputum or pulmonary functions or reduces morbidity and mortality. Exercise is not a replacement for regular physiotherapy in adults.[29] [30]

Bronchodilators

The indications for and use of bronchodilators in adults are identical to those in children.

Mucolytic agents

There is no evidence that traditional mucolytic agents have a role in the management of adults.

Corticosteroids

There is no primary role for corticosteroid treatment of the lung disease associated with cystic fibrosis in adults. Corticosteroid treatment given orally is indicated for the treatment of allergic bronchopulmonary aspergillosis and may be tried for continuing pulmonary deterioration despite aggressive antibiotic treatment. Inhaled corticosteroids are indicated for symptoms suggestive of asthma.

21

Nutrition

The attainment of normal growth in children is associated with less severe pulmonary disease. Adults with chronic pulmonary infection may have sufficient weight loss to lead to frank cachexia. This may be caused in part by increased energy expenditure secondary to the basic gene defect; in part by the increased work of breathing; and in part by the host's metabolic response to injury and infection in the lungs.[31 32] Adequate attention to nutrition is essential in the care of adults and their pulmonary problems (see chapter 7).

Complications of lung disease

Pneumothorax

There is a 1% annual incidence of spontaneous pneumothorax and up to 10% of patients will eventually have one. Pneumothorax is no longer considered to be a poor prognostic factor.[33] The outcome of an episode depends on background lung function, which governs the tolerance of the pneumothorax. Survival after the first pneumothorax is roughly 30 months with a 50%–70% chance of recurrence.[34] Signs and symptoms usually include pain, tachypnoea, tachycardia, dyspnoea, pallor and cyanosis. Tube drainage is needed when 15%–20% of a hemithorax is involved and there is respiratory distress. For smaller pneumothoraces observation in hospital may be sufficient, though needle aspiration should be considered.

Occasionally the pneumothorax fails to resolve even after a period of suction, and more invasive approaches such as chemical pleurodesis, limited surgical pleurodesis, partial pleurectomy, and oversewing or stapling of subpleural blebs may be needed. When deciding on such treatment it is important to consider the future potential of the patient for heart-lung transplantation (see chapter 8). Generally, chemical pleurodesis is reserved for those patients who are in poor clinical condition and who are not being considered for future transplantation. For many patients the benefits of surgery greatly outway the risks. Partial pleurectomy is highly successful but this option, as with any surgical intervention, should be discussed with a transplant centre if the patient is eligible for such treatment. For recurrent pneumothoraces surgery remains the best option. The effectiveness of interventions such as thoracoscopy with carbon dioxide laser ablation and stapling of blebs remains to be confirmed.

Haemoptysis

This varies from minor streaking of the sputum, quite common in adults, to recurrent heavy haemoptysis. The registry data of the United States Cystic Fibrosis Foundation indicate that about 1% of patients have a major haemoptysis each year. Haemoptyses are often associated with exacerbations of pulmonary symptoms which require intravenous treatment with antibiotics. Antibiotic treatment combined with admission to hospital and gentle physiotherapy is usually enough to settle such episodes.

Persistent or severe haemoptyses may necessitate bronchoscopy to identify the source of the blood loss. Once identified, bleeding can be stopped by embolisation of the bronchial artery, though this is a potentially hazardous procedure and requires an experienced specialist radiologist.[35] If bleeding persists and bronchial artery embolisation is not available or fails, local pulmonary resection should be considered. If appropriate this decision should be discussed with a transplant centre. In the later stages of lung disease severe haemoptysis may require palliative management only.

Respiratory failure

In the later phases of pulmonary disease patients may develop intermittent respiratory failure. Many progress to chronic hypoxaemia, and eventually develop type II respiratory failure and cor pulmonale.

Treatment is essentially palliative and consists of responding to exacerbations of symptoms and type II respiratory failure with antibiotics, supplementary low dose oxygen (24%–28%), diuretics, and digoxin. Nocturnal oxygen supplementation improves general wellbeing and may reduce the number of hospital admissions, but its efficacy remains controversial. The use of long term oxygen treatment is based on the beneficial effects reported in chronic obstructive airways disease, but no improvement in mortality, morbidity or exercise tolerance has been shown in patients with cystic fibrosis, though the improved quality of sleep during oxygen treatment may allow some patients to continue at work or at school.[36]

The use of assisted ventilation in patients with end stage lung disease is a controversial issue. Generally ventilation is not

23

recommended though nasal intermittent positive pressure ventilation gives short to medium term support for patients awaiting heart-lung transplantation.[37]

New and future treatments

Amiloride, adenosine triphosphate (ATP) and uridine triphosphate (UTP)

Amiloride given by aerosol inhibits absorption of sodium by the epithelial cells in the airways. Treatment reduces sputum viscosity, the loss of FEV_1 and forced vital capacity (FVC), and increases mucociliary and cough clearances.[38 39] Amiloride has the disadvantages of having to be given four times a day by nebuliser. Larger trials to find out its efficacy are underway.

The nucleotides ATP and UTP increase chloride efflux from epithelial cells in the respiratory tract. As with amiloride this effect occurs at the apical surface, hence the potential for nebulised treatment, particularly when these agents are combined with amiloride.[40] The role for this type of treatment is currently unknown but clinical trials have started.

DNase

A major factor that increases the viscosity of sputum is DNA derived from the host's inflammatory cells. Recombinant human DNase 1 (rhDNase 1) in aerosol form, which cleaves extracellular DNA, is beneficial, safe, and biochemically active in adult patients.[41, 42] Both FEV_1 and FVC improved after one week and 10 days treatment compared with baseline values.[42 43] Ten days treatment produced a mean increase of 13.3% in FEV_1 at a lower

---

Newer and future treatments in cystic fibrosis

- Nebulised amiloride
- Nebulised nucleotides (ATP & UTP)
- Nebulised DNase
- Ibuprofen (or other NSAIDs)
- Pentoxifylline (or other xanthines)
- α1-anti-proteinase
- SL PI
- Antielastases
- Gene therapy

---

dose than earlier studies (2.5 mg twice daily).[43]

A placebo controlled study of 24 weeks' treatment with either 2.5 mg once or twice daily in 968 adults and children confirmed modest benefits in lung function. Compared with placebo, both dosage regimens reduced the number of exacerbations by 28%–37% and there was increased sense of overall wellbeing.[44]

Anti-inflammatory agents

Anti-inflammatory agents may have a role in cystic fibrosis by suppressing the host's inflammatory response. Preliminary results of a trial in 85 children and adults taking high dose ibuprofen, a broad spectrum non-steroidal anti-inflammatory agent, indicate preservation of lung function over a four year treatment period in mild lung disease.[45] Compounds capable of specifically antagonising proteases, such as α_1-antitrypsin,[46] serum leucocyte proteinase inhibitor (SLPI),[47] and ICI-200, 800 have been studied. There may be other agents in the future, such as humanised monoclonal antibodies to, or receptor blocking agents for, cytokines and other mediators. Possibly agents already available such as pentoxifylline (which down-regulates ex-vivo neutrophil function) may have a role.[48]

Anti-elastases are potentially a useful treatment. Nebulised human α_1-antitrypsin changes the protease/antiprotease balance in the fluid lining the pulmonary epithelium in favour of anti-proteolysis. Seven days' treatment produced effective antielastase activity in the airways.[46] Nebulised recombinant SLPI increased *in vivo* antineutrophil elastase activity and neutralised active proteolytic enzymes.[47]

Gene treatment

Gene treatment is considered to be the ultimate treatment goal for lung disease in cystic fibrosis. A correct copy of the cystic fibrosis transmembrane conductance regulator (CFTR) gene can be delivered to respiratory epithelial cells using adenoviruses or liposome vectors.[49-57] There remain many unanswered major technical, clinical, and ethical questions about this form of treatment. Early studies of the safety of gene transfer using "designer" virus and liposome treatment have started in the United States and Great Britain.[51-57] Successful transfer of the CFTR gene into the nose using an adenovirus was reported in three patients.[55]

25

This led to gene expression, CFTR production, and correction of the nasal potential difference. Some of these changes lasted for 21 days. In a further study in which CFTR was delivered by adenovirus to the nose and lungs, mRNA and CFTR protein were detected in the nose of one patient, and CFTR protein in the bronchial epithelium of another.[56] Unfortunately, the large number of viral particles caused airways inflammation in another patient. Liposome-mediated CFTR gene transfer has been reported successfully in mice with cystic fibrosis.[49 50] A single report of the same method used in human noses indicated successful gene transfer with partial correction of the CFTR deficit over a seven day period.[57] There was evidence of gene incorporation or mRNA product in most of the nine treated subjects. This suggests that liposomal-mediated gene transfer is possible, but at present the efficiency of gene delivery is low and further development is needed.[57] Within the next decade trials leading to successful gene treatment can be expected.

Organisation of care for adults with cystic fibrosis

There is a consensus that specialised management centres are the ideal for the care of both children and adults with cystic fibrosis.[58 59] Such centres are being developed worldwide for adult patients and the core is usually a team including a physician, often a specialist in respiratory diseases, specialist nurses, physiotherapists, dietitians, a psychologist, and social workers (box). Such an approach results in improved survival over care in non-specialist centres.[60] Such centres care for all aspects of cystic fibrosis, either alone or sharing care with non-centre hospitals and general practitioners. Centralised care has the potential benefits of enhancing research into treatment and care, maintaining the throughput of appropriate patients to heart-lung transplantation centres, and providing a terminal care and bereavement service. Care in a specialist centre was also favoured by patients who received a more intensive pattern of care.[61] Various levels of care can be offered depending on size of the patient population, local expertise, and enthusiasm (box). Clearly an integrated shared pattern of support and care could be based on these levels to provide for input from general practice to national specialist centres.

26

The team for managing adult cystic fibrosis and its complications

General team:	Experts required for advice on managing complications:
Consultant chest physician(s)	
Back-up physician in adult cystic fibrosis	Endocrinologist/diabetologist
Clinical nurse specialist(s)	Gastroenterologist
Specialist physiotherapists for inpatient and outpatient care	General surgeon
	Anaesthetist
Specialist dietitian	Ear, nose and throat surgeon
Social worker	Clinical geneticist
Pharmacist(s)	Obstetrician/gynaecologist
Medical microbiologist	Thoracic surgeon
Chaplain/religious advisor	Rheumatologist

Adult patients need to consider career and employment prospects in the light of the severity of their cystic fibrosis and its complications. With help from health professionals they need to make an assessment of their current and future health so that appropriate type of employment can be undertaken. A survey of 860 adults with cystic fibrosis showed that 54% were employed, 14% were students, and only 24% were unemployed because of ill health.[62] An important issue that often comes to the fore at the time of seeking employment is whether to tell a prospective employer about the condition, which really needs to be considered in each case.

An area of difficulty is independent living. Even with reasonable employment adults with cystic fibrosis seem to have difficulty, with 56% of men and 48% of women living at home with their parents.[62] Parental concern and involvement makes independent housing difficult for such patients and is compounded by the difficulty of obtaining life insurance, loans, or mortgages. It may be that for adults who require independence from their parents, special needs accommodation may have to be sought and a specialist social worker is needed to provide assistance.

The development of normal adult relationships is made more difficult by the impact of cystic fibrosis. There are various reasons for this (see chapter 9), but men have more difficulty than women in developing partnerships and may need considerable counselling and help with these problems. Among people who do not have cystic fibrosis 61% of adults are married or cohabiting compared

Levels of care in cystic fibrosis

Level one
National specialist centre
Provides care for hundreds of patients including the most severely ill. Acts as a national resource for all doctors and patients, and provides national education and training. Provides major research facilities and is able to coordinate national multicentre trials.

Level two
Regional specialist centre
Provides care for over 100 patients with special weekly cystic fibrosis clinics. Acts as a training, resource, and research centre with specialist doctors and paramedical staff.

Level three
Local specialist/large district centre
Provides service to around 50 patients from one to three districts. May be a special clinic with some specialist interest among clinicians and paramedical staff. Care may be shared with a level one or two centre.

Level four
Local district general hospital
Provides day-to-day medical care for about 5–10 patients. Patients usually seen on the ward or in general clinics. Most patients also attend a level two or level three hospital.

Level five
General practitioner or community care
General Practitioner involvement varies from writing repeat prescriptions for medication to full participation in home programmes. Local community units generally do not provide specialist services and community support is provided by a specialist cystic fibrosis centre.

with only 34% of those with cystic fibrosis. Of women with cystic fibrosis 44% are living with a partner while only 26% of men are in a similar relationship. Clearly adult patients need practical and professional support from the multidisciplinary team with regard to these aspects of life.

Care for adults with cystic fibrosis requires an interdisciplinary approach to a multisystem disorder. Over the last 30 years there has been a pronounced increase in life expectancy, and over the next decade an increasing proportion of patients will be adults. For patients born in 1990 the likely median survival is estimated at 40 years, which indicates a need for the care of adult patients for several decades to come.[1]

References

1 Means MB. Cystic fibrosis: the first 50 years. A review of the clinical problems and their management. In: Dodge JA, Brock DJH, Widdicombe JH, eds. *Cystic fibrosis: current topics*. Vol 1. Chichester: John Wiley, 1993: 217–50.
2 Hodson ME, Beldon I, Power R, Duncan FR, Bamber M, Batten JC. Sweat tests to diagnose cystic fibrosis in adults. *BMJ* 1983; **286**: 1381–2.
3 Chrispin A, Norman A. The systematic evaluation of the chest radiograph in cystic fibrosis. *Pediatr Radiol* 1974; **2**: 101–6.
4 Brasfield D, Hicks G, Soong S-J, Tiller RE. The chest roentgenogram in cystic fibrosis: a new scoring system. *Pediatrics* 1979; **63**: 24–9.
5 Conway SP, Pond MN, Bowler I, Smith DL, Simmonds EJ, Joanes DN. The chest radiograph in cystic fibrosis: a new scoring system compared with the Chrispin-Norman and Brasfield scores. *Thorax* 1994; **49**: 860–2.
6 Lynch DA, Brasch RC, Hardy MKA, Webb WR. Paediatric pulmonary disease: assessment with high-resolution ultrafast CT. *Radiology* 1990; **176**: 243–8.
7 Bhalla M, Turcios N, Aponte V, *et al.* Cystic fibrosis: scoring system with thin-section. *Radiology* 1991; **179**: 783–8.
8 Høiby N, Pedersen SS. Estimated risk of cross-infection with *Pseudomonas aeruginosa* in Danish cystic fibrosis patients. *Acta Paediatrica Scandinavica* 1989; **78**: 395–404.
9 Tummler B, Koopmann U, Grothees D, Weissbrodt H, Steinkamp G, Vonderhardt H. Nosocomial acquisition of *Pseudomonas aeruginosa* by cystic fibrosis patients. *J Clin Microbiol* 1991; **29**: 1265–7.
10 Valerius N, Koch C, Høiby N. Prevention of chronic *Pseudomonas aeruginosa* colonisation in cystic fibrosis by early treatment. *Lancet* 1991; **338**: 725–6.
11 Pedersen SS, Jensen T, Høiby N, Koch C, Flensborg EW. Management of *Pseudomonas aeruginosa* lung infection in Danish cystic fibrosis patients. *Acta Paediatrica Scandinavica* 1987; **76**: 955–61.
12 Rayner RJ, Wiseman MS, Cordon SM, Norman D, Hiller EJ, Shale DJ. Inflammatory markers in cystic fibrosis. *Respir Med* 1991; **85**: 139–45.
13 Norman D, Elborn JS, Cordon SM *et al.* Plasma tumour necrosis factor-α in cystic fibrosis. *Thorax* 1991; **46**: 91–5.
14 Regelmann WE, Elliott GR, Warwick WJ, Clawson CC. Reduction of sputum *Pseudomonas aeruginosa* densely by antibiotics improves lung function in cystic fibrosis more than bronchodilators and chest physiotherapy alone. *Am Rev Respir Dis* 1990; **141**: 914–21.
15 Smith A. Antibiotic resistance is not relevant in infections in cystic fibrosis. *Ped Pulmonol* 1990; **5** (suppl): 93.
16 Ramsey B, Smith A, Williams-Warren J. The efficacy of aerosolized tobramycin administration in cystic fibrosis patients: results of a multi-centre, placebo controlled, cross-over trial. *Ped Pulmonol* 1991; **6** (suppl): 7A.
17 Jensen T, Pedersen SS, Garne S, Heilmann C, Høiby N, Koch C. Colistin inhalation therapy in cystic fibrosis patients with chronic *Pseudomonas aeruginosa* lung infection. *J Antimicrob Chemother* 1987; **19**: 831–8.
18 Nir M, Johansen HK, Høiby N. Low incidence of pulmonary *Pseudomonas cepacia* infection in Danish cystic fibrosis patients. *Acta Paediatr* 1992; **81**: 1042–3.
19 Editorial. *Pseudomonas cepacia* – more than a harmless commensal? Lancet 1992; **339**: 1385–6.
20 FitzSimmons SC. The changing epidemiology of cystic fibrosis. *J Pediatr* 1993; **122**: 1–9.

21 Thomassen MJ, Demko CA, Doershuk CF, Stern RC, Klinger JD. *Pseudomonas cepacia*: decrease in colonization in patients with cystic fibrosis. *Am Rev Respir Dis* 1986; **134**: 669–71.

22 Govan JWR, Brown PH, Maddison J *et al.* Evidence for transmission of *Pseudomonas cepacia* by social contact in cystic fibrosis. *Lancet* 1993; **342**: 15–19.

23 Döring G, Shaffar L, eds. *Epidemiology of pulmonary infections by Pseudomonas in patients with cystic fibrosis: a consensus report.* Paris: Association Française de Lutte contre la Mucoviscidose, French Cystic Fibrosis Association, 1993.

24 *Cystic Fibrosis Statement on Pseudomonas Cepacia.* London: Cystic Fibrosis Trust for Great Britain, 1993.

25 Isles A, Maclusky I, Corey M *et al. Pseudomonas cepacia* infection in cystic fibrosis: an emerging problem. *J Pediatr* 1984; **104**: 206–10.

26 Lewin LO, Byard PJ, Davis PB. Effects of *Pseudomonas cepacia* colonization on survival and pulmonary function of cystic fibrosis patients. *J Clin Epidemiol* 1909; **43**: 125–31.

27 Tomashefski JF Jr, Thomasse MJ, Bruce MC, Goldberg HI, Konstan MW, Stern RC. *Pseudomonas cepacia* associated pneumonia in cystic fibrosis. *Arch Pathol Lab Med* 1988; **112**: 166–72.

28 Nelson JW, Doherty CJ, Brown PH, Greening AP, Kaufmann ME, Govan JRW. *Pseudomonas cepacia* in inpatients with cystic fibrosis. *Lancet* 1991; **338**: 1525.

29 Zach M, Oberwaldner B, Hauser F. Cystic fibrosis: physical exercise versus chest physiotherapy. *Arch Dis Child* 1982; **57**: 587–9.

30 Orenstein D, Franklin B, Doershuk C *et al.* Exercise conditioning and cardiopulmonary fitness in cystic fibrosis. *Chest* 1981; **80**: 392–8.

31 O'Rawe A, McIntosh I, Dodge JA *et al.* Increased energy expenditure in cystic fibrosis is associated with specific mutations. *Clin Sci* 1992; **82**: 71–6.

32 Elborn JS, Cordon SM, Western PJ, Macdonald IA, Shale DJ. Tumour necrosis factor-α, resting energy expenditure and cachexia in cystic fibrosis. *Clin Sci* 1993; **85**: 563–8.

33 Seddon D, Hodson M. Surgical management of pneumothorax in cystic fibrosis. *Thorax* 1988; **43**: 739–40.

34 Spector M, Stern R. Pneumothorax in cystic fibrosis: a 26-year experience. *Ann Thorac Surg* 1989; **47**: 204–7.

35 Sweeney N, Fellows K. Bronchial artery embolisation for severe haemoptysis in cystic fibrosis. *Chest* 1990; **97**: 1322–6.

36 Coates A. Oxygen therapy, exercise and cystic fibrosis. *Chest* 1992; **101**: 2–4.

37 Hodson ME, Madden BP, Steven MH, Tsang VT, Yacoub MH. Non-invasive mechanical ventilation for cystic fibrosis patients – a potential bridge to transplantation. *Eur Resp J* 1991; **4**: 524–7.

38 Knowles MR, Church NL, Waltner WE *et al.* A pilot study of aerosolized amiloride for the treatment of lung disease in cystic fibrosis. *N Engl J Med* 1990; **322**: 1189–94.

39 Tomkiewicz RP, App EM, Zayas JG *et al.* Amiloride inhalation therapy in cystic fibrosis: influence on ion content, hydration and rheology of sputum. *Am Rev Respir Dis* 1993; **148**: 1002–7.

40 Knowles MR, Clark LL, Boucher RC. Activation by extracellular nucleotides of chloride secretion in the airway epithelium of patients with cystic fibrosis. *N Engl J Med* 1991; **325**: 533–8.

41 Aitken ML, Burke W, McDonald G, Shak S, Montgomery AB, Smith A. Recombinant human DNase inhalation in normal and cystic fibrosis subjects: a phase I study. *JAMA* 1992; **267**: 1947–51.

42 Hubbard RC, McElvaney NG, Birrer P *et al.* A preliminary study of aerosolised recombinant human deoxyribose I in the sputum of cystic fibrosis. *N Engl J Med* 1992; **326**: 812–15.

43 Ranasinha C, Assoufi B, Shak S *et al.* Efficacy and safety of short-term

administration of aerosolised recombinant human DNase I in adults with stable stage cystic fibrosis. *Lancet* 1993; **342**: 199–202.

44 Fuchs HJ, Borowitz DS, Christiansen DH *et al.* Effect of aerosolised recombinant human DNase on exacerbations of respiratory symptoms and on pulmonary function in patients with cystic fibrosis. *N Engl J Med* 1994; **331**: 637–42.

45 Konstan MW, Byard PJ, Hoppel CL, Davis PB. Effect of high-dose ibuprofen in patients with cystic fibrosis. *N Engl J Med* 1995; **332**: 848–54.

46 McElvaney NG, Hubbard RC, Birrer P *et al.* Aerosol α_1-antitrypsin treatment for cystic fibrosis. *Lancet* 1991; **337**: 392–4.

47 McElvaney NG, Doujaiji B, Moan MJ, Burnham MR, Wu MC, Crystal RG. Pharmacokinetics of recombinant secretory leukoprotease inhibitor aerosolised to normals and individuals with cystic fibrosis. *Am Rev Respir Dis* 1993; **148**: 1056–60.

48 Slater K, Wiseman MS, Shale DJ, Fletcher J. The effect of pentoxifylline on neutrophil function *in vivo* and *ex vivo* in human volunteers. In: Mansell GL, Novick WJ, eds. *Pentoxifylline and leukocyte function.* New Jersey: Hoechst-Roussel Ltd, 1988; 115–23.

49 Hyde SC, Gill DR, Higgins CF, *et al.* Correction of the ion transport defect in cystic fibrosis transgenic mice by gene therapy. *Nature* 1993; **362**: 250–5.

50 Alton EWFW. Non-invasive liposome-mediated gene delivery can correct the ion transport defect in cystic fibrosis mutant mice. *Nature Genetics* 1993; **5**: 135–42.

51 Rosenfeld MA, Yoshimura K, Trapnell BC *et al.* *In vivo* transfer of human cystic fibrosis transmembrane conductance regulator gene to airway epithelium. *Cell* 1992; **68**: 143–55.

52 Brody SL, Crystal RG. Adenovirus-mediated *in vivo* gene transfer. *Annals of the New York Academy of Sciences* 1994; **716**: 90–101.

53 Welsh MJ, Smith AE, Zabner J *et al.* Clinical protocol. Cystic fibrosis gene therapy using adenovirus vector: *in vivo* safety and efficacy in nasal epithelium. *Hum Gene Ther* 1994; **5**: 209–19.

54 Boucher RC, Knowles MR, Johnson LG *et al.* Gene therapy for cystic fibrosis using E1 adenovirus: a Phase 1 trial in the nasal cavity. *Hum Gene Ther* 1994; **5**: 615–39.

55 Zabner J, Conture LA, Gregory RJ, Graham SM, Smith AE, Welsh MJ. Adenovirus mediated gene transfer transiently corrects the chloride transport defect in nasal epithelium of patients with cystic fibrosis. *Cell* 1993; **75**: 207–16.

56 Crystal RG, McElvaney NG, Rosenfeld MA *et al.* Administration of an adenovirus containing the human CFTR cDNA to the respiratory tract of individuals with cystic fibrosis. *Nature Genetics* 1994; **8**: 42–51.

57 Caplen NJ, Alton EWFW, Middleton PG *et al.* Liposome-mediated CFTR gene transfer to the nasal epithelium of patients with cystic fibrosis. *Nature Medicine* 1995; **1**: 39–46.

58 Royal College of Physicians. *Cystic fibrosis in adults; recommendations for the care of adults in the United Kingdom.* London: RCGP, 1990.

59 Clinic Standards Advisory Group. *Cystic fibrosis: access to and availability of specialist services.* London: HMSO, 1993.

60. Corey M, McLaughlin FJ, Williams M, Levison H. A comparison of survival, growth and pulmonary function in patients with cystic fibrosis in Boston and Toronto. *J Clin Epidemiol* 1988; **41**: 585–91.

61 Walters SJ, Britton J, Hodson ME. Hospital care for adults with cystic fibrosis: an overview and comparison between special cystic fibrosis clinics and general clinics using a patient questionnaire. *Thorax* 1994; **49**: 300–6.

62 Walters SJ, Hodson ME. Demographic and social characteristics of adults with cystic fibrosis in the United Kingdom. *BMJ* 1993; **306**: 549–52.

3 Experimental work in mice

JULIA R DORIN, DAVID J PORTEOUS

Remarkable progress has been made in the biochemical understanding of cystic fibrosis in the six years since the cystic fibrosis transmembrane conductance regulator (CFTR) gene was cloned. Nevertheless important gaps remain in our understanding of the pathophysiology of this complex disorder. Progress has always been frustrated by the limited availability of clinical material from affected tissues at critical stages in the development of the disease. Help has come in the last three years with the advent of murine models for the disease engineered by targeted mutagenesis of the murine CFTR gene.[1-4]

Cystic fibrosis in mice: how and why

An animal model which accurately reflects a clinical disease is essential for an understanding of the pathophysiology of the disorder and for planning and testing new treatments. There is no known natural animal model of cystic fibrosis. Laboratory mice are widely used to study mammalian development and have provided models for human disorders. There are important similarities between the human and murine CTFR gene[5 6] (Table 3.1), which suggest that the function of the gene is conserved between the species. Cystic fibrosis is characterised by defective chloride ion transport,[7] so it is relevant that wild-type mice and normal human subjects have similar bioelectric properties in both the respiratory and intestinal tracts consistent with a common mechanism of cAMP-dependent chloride ion conductance.[8]

Table 3.1   CFTR conservation between mouse and man

	amino acid identity (%)	amino acid similarity (%)
Whole protein	78	89
First nucleotide binding domain	81	94
Exon 10	86	98
R domain	69	81
Second nucleotide binding domain	84	94
Of 133 missense mutations in man	92	99

Cystic fibrosis has a recessive mode of inheritance, so the first step towards modelling required identification and then inactivation of the homologous gene. This is only technically possible in laboratory mice, as outlined in Figure 3.1. There are two essential components to this technique. Firstly, it is necessary to have the ability to culture cells from the inner cell mass of the early murine embryo, to manipulate these in culture, and to reimplant them into donor blastocysts and thereby generate chimeric mice comprising a mixture of cells from the donor and recipient blastocyst. Secondly, it is necessary to engineer a precise alteration in the chosen gene in the cultured mouse embryonal stem cells, using either "gene targeting" or gene "knockout" methods. There are essentially two ways of introducing mutations into the CFTR or any other chosen gene in mouse embryonal stem cells. A single recombination event can be used to insert an additional fragment of DNA into the targeted gene to disrupt its function (referred to as insertional gene targeting). Alternatively a double reciprocal recombination event can be used to delete a vital segment of the gene (referred to as gene replacement). Gene targeting therefore relies on a homologous recombination event between the chromosomal locus and genomic fragments cloned into the targeting vector (Figure 3.1). Homologous recombination is the exception rather than the rule in mammalian cells; the rare gene targeting event must be identified against a background of random integration events. This is made possible by incorporating selectable markers into the targeting vector and screening transfected embryonal stem clones individually for the presence of precise, predicted changes in the structure of the targeted locus.

The four groups who have so far been successful in disrupting the murine Cftr gene and generating cystic fibrosis "knockout" mice have used both gene targeting strategies (insertion or replacement) and two different regions of the gene (exon 3 or 10).

33

The designation of the Cftr mutant alleles follow the nomenclature recommendations of the Committee on Standardised Genetic Nomenclature for Mice and use abbreviations of the laboratory in which they were derived (UNC, HGU, Cam and Bay). Variations in the targeting strategies used by the four groups have affected the phenotypic outcome. The mice created at the University of North Carolina (UNC),[1] the MRC Human Genetics Unit, Edinburgh (HGU),[2] and the Wellcome Institute, Cambridge (CAM),[3] have disruptions of exon 10 denoted cftr^{m1UNC}, cftr^{m1HGU}, and cftr^{m1Cam} respectively. The group at Baylor College of Medicine targeted exon 3 (cftr^{m1Bay}). The Cftr^{m1UNC} and Cftr^{m1Cam} mutant mice were produced in a similar way by the positive negative selection "replacement" gene targeting scheme.[9] Correct gene targeting occurs through a double reciprocal exchange between homologous gene and vector sequences. As a consequence, the region of the endogenous gene that lies between the crossovers is replaced, there is no molecular mechanism for reversion to wild type, and the mutations are absolute "nulls". Hence, these mice are phenotypically indistinguishable and can be considered synonymous for this discussion. Dorin et al[2] and O'Neal et al[4] have both described insertional gene targeting strategies into exon 10 (Cftr^{m1HGU}) or exon 3 (Cftr^{m1Bay}), respectively. Insertion into the genomic target occurs without loss of sequence and aberrant splicing around insertional mutations can in some instances result in wild type mRNA. While the Hprt insertional gene disruptions have been shown to be absolute "nulls" under stringent biochemical selection,[10] an insertional disruption of N-myc was found to be "leaky".[11]

It is not possible to detect Cftr mRNA in the exon 10 cftr^{m1UNC} or the cftr^{m1CAM} replacement mice[1] (W. Colledge, personal communication), or in the cftr^{m1Bay} exon 3 insertional mutant animals.[4] By contrast, the cftr^{m1HGU} homozygotes display a low level of wild type Cftr mRNA which is the result of aberrant splicing and exon skipping.[12] Perhaps the efficiency of alternative splicing in the exon 3 region of the Cftr gene is low compared with the exon 10 region, and this explains why the Cftr^{m1HGU} insertion is slightly "leaky" and the Cftr^{m1Bay} insertion is not. Interestingly, alternative splicing occurs in regions adjacent to exon 10 in the CFTR gene (exon 11b in mice[13] and exon 9 in humans).[14] The fact that the cftr^{m1HGU} mutation is on an outbred background whereas the cftr^{m1Bay} mutation is on an inbred background may also influence the efficiency with which exon skipping occurs.

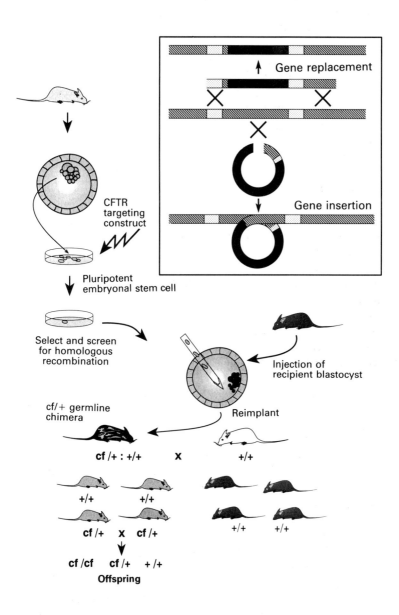

Electrophysiology

As predicted, all four murine models have an electrophysiological phenotype consistent with CFTR dysfunction and can be distinguished from wild type animals by defective chloride ion transport.[2 4 15 16] We have discussed the comparison of the different mice with each other and with humans in detail elsewhere,[17] and this is the subject of chapter four, but just how closely the four cystic fibrosis murine models reproduce the bioelectric properties seen in subjects with cystic fibrosis can be seen from the summary shown in Table 3.2.

In the intestine of cftr^{m1HGU} mice[17] (Smith *et al*, unpublished observations) and the cftr^{m1UNC} mutant homozygotes,[18] cAMP-activated chloride transport is reduced and as expected calcium-mediated chloride conductance is also reduced. In the pancreas and the respiratory tract, in common with humans, the cAMP-activated, but not the calcium-activated, chloride ion transport is reduced.[17,18,19] In the murine pancreas the calcium-mediated chloride ion transport is an order of magnitude larger than that observed in humans and is likely to play a greater part in maintaining pancreatic fluid balance in mice than it does in humans, where CFTR activity is a major determinant (Table 3.3). This channel may be upregulated in the pancreas of the cftr^{m1UNC} mice.[18] Together with the species difference of relative channel activities, this may explain the lack of pancreatic disease in all the cf/cf mice.[1 2 4 16] An additional electrophysiological difference between mice and humans is the reduced sodium absorption in the tracheas of cf/cf mice,[17 20] whereas in patients with cystic fibrosis

---

Figure 3.1 This general strategy for creating a mouse model for cystic fibrosis by gene targeting in embryonal stem cells begins with cells from an inbred mouse strain that carry a coat colour mutation[a] (light colour). The embryonal stem cells are cultured and modified either by insertional or replacement gene targeting and cells that have the desired CFTR alteration are identified and reintroduced into the blastocoel cavity of a blastocyst of a different (dark) coat colour genotype. If the cells are totipotent they will contribute to all tissues of the developing mouse including the germline. Cells that colonised the skin display the coat colour that was derived from the embryonal stem cells (light) on a dark background (host blastocyst) and therefore have cells which are either +/+ or cf/+. Chimeras are tested for germline transmission by mating to mice that will allow detection of the embryonal stem cell coat colour mutations. Half of the offspring derived from the embryonal stem cells will carry the gene targeted chromosome and these are identified by DNA analysis. Mating of heterozygous cf/+ mice results in the production of cf/cf homozygotes.

Table 3.2   Comparison of cystic fibrosis phenotypes in man and mouse – residual CFTR function

Species	Allele	Nature of mutation	Residual CFTR function
Humans	R347P R117H R334W	Missense Arg to "other" in first membrane spanning domain	~33%, ~15% } of wild type ~4%
Humans	ΔF508	3 bp Deletion resulting in loss of a Phe residue in exon 10 of first nucleotide binding domain	Functional if correctly localised, but not detectable *in vivo*
Mouse	cftr^m1UNC and cftr^m1Cam	Disruption of chromosomal exon 10 by replacement gene targeting	None detectable
Mouse	cftr^m1Bay	Duplication of exon 3 by insertional gene targeting	None detectable
Mouse	cftr^m1HGU	Insertional gene targeting into exon 10	<10% of normal amount of CFTR mRNA produced by aberrant splicing

this tissue displays increased sodium absorption.[21 22] Finally two species differences in the cellular composition of the respiratory tract in humans and mice are perhaps noteworthy. Mice have a relative paucity of submucosal glands and in humans these glands have been shown to be the major site of CFTR gene expression in the lung, and one of the first sites of histological abnormality.[23 24] Additionally, the distribution of cells in the tracheal epithelium of mice is significantly different from that in humans with 50%–60% of the cellular component being Clara cells, which are not a prominent feature in man. The extent of lung disease in the cf/cf mice will lead us to question the importance of these differences in disease involvement.

In summary, the characteristic defect in cAMP-mediated chloride secretion is present throughout the respiratory and intestinal tracts in each of the murine models. Furthermore, many of the other associated abnormalities of ion transport found in humans are also seen, with the exception of increased sodium absorption in the trachea. This suggests that these models will be of value in furthering the understanding of the pathophysiology of cystic fibrosis and in studying the effects of novel treatments.

Table 3.3 Comparison of the bioelectric phenotype of cystic fibrosis respiratory and gastrointestinal tracts in humans and mice

Tissue	Measurement	Humans	Mice
Nasal epithelium	Baseline PD	⇑	⇑
	Sodium absorption	⇑	⇑
	cAMP mediated chloride conductance	⇓	⇓
	Calcium related chloride conductance	Preserved	Preserved
Lower respiratory tract	Baseline PD	Preserved or ⇑	Preserved or ⇓
	Sodium absorption	⇑	⇓
	cAMP mediated chloride conductance	⇓	⇓ or Preserved
	Calcium related chloride conductance	Preserved	Preserved
Gastro-intestinal tract	Baseline PD	⇓ or Preserved	⇓ or Preserved
	cAMP mediated chloride conductance	⇓	⇓
	Calcium related chloride conductance	⇓	⇓
	Sodium-glucose cotransport	⇑	Preserved

Histopathology of mice with cystic fibrosis

Intestinal Disease

Table 3.4 describes the long term survival of mice with cystic fibrosis from the four different groups. The phenotype of the mice produced by Dorin et al[2] is significantly different from that of the other three models.[1 3 4] These latter animals all have a severe phenotype in terms of the morbidity and mortality because of the severity of intestinal disease. Within one week of birth, 40%–80% present with severe bowel obstruction which leads to intestinal perforation, peritonitis, and death. A second critical period resulting in death is around weaning, leaving less than 5% of these mutant animals surviving into adulthood. The intestinal site of the

Table 3.4   Comparison of severity of intestinal disease in mice and humans

	Mice				Humans
Mutant allele	cftr^m1UNC	cftr^m1Cam	cftr^m1Bay	cftr^m1HGU	>300
Death within 1 week of birth	~50%	~80%	~40%	~5%	10%–20% Ileal blockage (meconium ileus) or obstruction in large intestine (meconium plug) in newborns
Death around weaning	~40%	~10%	~10%	~2%	Distal intestinal obstruction syndrome
Death after 40 days	Not reported	Not reported	Not reported	2%	In ~20% of children and adults
Body weight at weaning	Reduced 10%–50%	Reduced 50%	Reduced 70%	No reduction	Failure to thrive and reduced growth rate
Survival to adulthood	<5%	<10%	Not reported (≤50%)	~93%	Intestinal blockage and obstruction not fatal, due to surgical intervention

perinatal blockage is either immediately proximal or distal to the caecum.[4][16] The animals that die at weaning may have the constriction located in the small intestine, but it is more commonly in the large intestine.

Roughly 5%–10% of newborn infants with cystic fibrosis present with *meconium ileus* and this is practically diagnostic of the disease.[24] These babies fail to pass meconium and develop abdominal distension which may result in perforation and peritonitis. A few babies with cystic fibrosis have a meconium plug in the large intestine and meconium passage is delayed, but this feature is shared with several clinical entities. The intestinal disease of the "severe" cystic fibrosis mutant mice is therefore similar to that observed in these few extreme clinical cases. Interestingly, the phenotype of the cystic fibrosis mice produced by Dorin *et al*[2] closely resembles the severity of intestinal disease seen in man. Only 5% of the cftr^{m1HGU} homozygous animals die perinatally from gut blockage which, when present, is similar to that observed in the other cystic fibrosis mice.[12] A further 2% of cftr^{m1HGU} homozygotes die at weaning, so 93% of homozygous mutant animals survive to adulthood and 2% of these die from distal intestinal obstruction similar to that observed in patients with cystic fibrosis and termed *meconium ileus* equivalent or distal intestinal obstruction syndrome. The small amount of mRNA found in the exon 10 insertional model seems to be enough to result in clearance of meconium in 95% of animals perinatally and 90% of animals overall. All four of the cystic fibrosis mutant mice have been reported as having mucin accumulation with dilatation of the crypts and engorgement and increase of goblet cells.[1][2][4][16] These gut abnormalities are displayed in only three quarters of the cftr^{m1HGU} homozygote animals that survive weaning.

Pancreatic disease

In humans, about 85% of subjects with cystic fibrosis have pancreatic insufficiency from birth.[24] The pancreas is histologically abnormal in almost every case and is often virtually destroyed. In contrast, there is little if any evidence in the cystic fibrosis mice of consistent or overt pancreatic histology akin to that seen in human cystic fibrosis. One reason for this species difference could be the dominant role of calcium-regulated chloride flux in mice.[19] A second, additive factor could be that the normal level of Cftr expression in the pancreas is appreciably reduced in mice compared with humans.[25] The lack of pancreatic involvement evident even in the absolute "null" cystic fibrosis mice does, however, question the presumption that *meconium ileus* in babies with cystic fibrosis is primarily a consequence of pancreatic malfunction and shifts the focus of attention towards malabsorption in the gastrointestinal tract.

Lung disease

Almost all of the morbidity and mortality in patients with cystic fibrosis is caused by lung disease. Although no histological abnormalities are present at birth, submucosal gland hypertrophy and dilated acinal and duct lumens are evident before chronic infections are established. Mucin accumulation and small airway obstruction is generally thought to lead to bronchiolitis and chronic infection, and then extensive bronchiectasis. Infectious pathogens are commonly *Staphylococcus aureus* followed by *Pseudomonas aeruginosa*.[24] The submucosal glands of the proximal airways are the site of highest level CFTR expression in the respiratory tract in man[23] although moderate levels of expression occur in non-ciliated cells lining the most distal airways.[26] Otherwise, CFTR expression in the epithelial lung cells is extremely low, with only an estimated 1 copy/cell of CFTR mRNA.[27] It has been suggested that the submucosal gland is a likely initial site of the pathogenesis of disease and a primary target for treatment, although there is no reason why absolute levels of normal gene expression should correlate with the relative importance of different cell and tissue types in disease.[28] It is only the consequence of gene dysfunction which is really relevant, and this can be judged only by empirical observation and direct experimentation.

In common with humans, none of the cf/cf mice present with respiratory tract disease at birth. There are some consistent and therefore probably important minor abnormalities (Table 3.5). It is presumed that external factors contribute to the development of the pulmonary complications in humans. Unlike pancreatic disease, there are no good correlations between genotype and susceptibility to lung disease,[29] although there is a suggestion that the ΔF508 homozygotes and some ΔF508 compound heterozygotes have increased susceptibility to early colonisation by *Ps aeruginosa*.[30] As a result of the good long term survival of the exon 10 insertional mouse model, it should be possible to define which of many putative factors are necessary for the development of cystic fibrosis lung disease or which augment the progress of the

Table 3.5 Comparison of cystic fibrosis phenotypes in humans and mice – respiratory tract disease

Species	Allele	Respiratory tract
Humans		No histological abnormality at birth
		Dilated acinar and duct lumens in submucosal glands before chronic infections
	R117H	Submucosal gland and goblet cell hypertrophy into the distal airways
		Mucin accumulation and small airway obstruction leading to bronchiolectasis and chronic infection, then
		extensive bronchiectasis
Mice	ΔF508	Chronic infection usually with *Staph aureus* initially and subsequently *Ps aeruginosa*
	cftr^{m1UNC}	Atrophy of serous gland tissue in nasal dorsolateral sinuses
		Dilation of ducts in nasal mucosa and proximal trachea
		Goblet cell hyperplasia in proximal airways
Mice	cftr^{m1Cam}	No histological abnormality reported
Mice	cftr^{m1Bay}	Dilatation of acini
		Accumulation of material in mucosal glands of pharynx
Mice	cftr^{m1HGU}	Frank lung disease induced after repeated exposure to *Staph aureus* or *B cepacia*

disease.

In considering the cftr^{m1HGU} mouse as a model for studying susceptibility to lung disease, the finding of Sheppard et al,[31] that the R347P and R117H mutations retained about 30% and 15% of wild type chloride conductance values, respectively, may be relevant. R347P/ΔF508 or R117H/ΔF508 compound heterozygotes are predicted to retain about 15% or 7.5% of normal CFTR function, respectively. Such patients are still diagnosed as having cystic fibrosis and still develop severe lung disease although the pancreatic involvement is less. The residual level of cAMP-mediated chloride secretion in the cftr^{m1HGU} mouse is therefore directly comparable to that patients with cystic fibrosis and lung disease. We find that the cftr^{m1HGU} mutant animals (housed in a conventional animal house) do not display significant differences in lung histology to their littermates although there is a trend of increased bronchitis, mucin accumulation, focal atelectasis and bronchiectasis. Repeated exposure to cystic fibrosis bacterial pathogens triggers mucin hypersecretion and precipitates the development of severe lung disease in the mutants but not littermate controls. The response to the pathogen mimics the clinical picture in patients (Davidson et al, unpublished observations). There are good grounds therefore to suspect that further studies in cystic fibrosis mice will allow the complex relationship between the CFTR gene dysfunction and susceptibility to infectious inflammatory lung disease to be elucidated.

Refining the mouse models

The analysis of the existing murine models suggests three obvious directions through genetic crossing that can yield further information. The first is to compare the phenotype of each strain on a variety of inbred genetic backgrounds to find out whether secondary genetic factors can account for the variability in residual chloride ion conductance and disease phenotype in cftr^{m1HGU} mice, and, by extension, in patients with cystic fibrosis. The second is to compare the phenotype of compound heterozygotes between cftr^{m1HGU} mice and absolute "null" mice in which there will be a further 50% reduction in the amount of wild type CFTR from that seen in the cftr^{m1HGU} homozygotes. Finally, it will be of interest to study the effect of crossing the Cftr mutant mice with other "knockout" mice or spontaneous mutant strains defective in other aspects of ion transport, fluid balance, or the inflammatory response.

Clinically relevant mutations in the mouse

Creating clinically relevant mutations in the mouse provides the opportunity to compare genotype and phenotype relationships on a controlled genetic background. In addition certain pharmacological or gene therapy strategies may be relevant to a particular mutant protein. The ΔF508 mutation has been introduced into the mouse Cftr gene by two gene targeting groups.[32][33] Two different strategies were employed, replacement and "hit and run".[34][35][36] In the replacement strategy used by Colledge et al,[32] the mouse exon 10 was replaced with an exon 10 containing a 3 base bair deletion to remove the phenylalanine codon and mimic ΔF508. The selection cassette was located in intron 10 so as not to interfere with correct Cftr gene expression. However, although ΔF508 mutant protein is made in the mice derived from these cells, the expression is reduced to about 15% of normal levels. The phenotype is essentially identical to the "null" mice with a high level of death from intestinal obstruction, but a question mark remains over whether the phenotype is affected by the very low level of mutant ΔF508 protein. An alternative strategy was used by van Doorninck et al,[33] where an insertional vector containing the ΔF508 mutation was used. The targeting vector encoded both positive and negative selection cassettes. After correctly targeted clones ("hits") were identified, the negative selection was applied and only clones which had lost vector sequence because of intrachromosomal recombination ("runs") survived. The genome can either revert to wild type sequence or will be modified to include the introduced mutation depending on whether the recombination event occurs proximal or distal to the modified site. Transcription from this mutant allele should be normal as the gene is only modified by the introduced mutation and vector sequences not present. Interestingly, these mice appear to have residual CFTR activity in terms of the forskolin response and show distended glands and goblet cell hypertrophy in the gut, but do not die from intestinal blockage.

Delaney et al[37] have produced mice carrying the G551D mutation thought to carry a reduced incidence of meconium ileus[38] in humans. The mutation was introduced into exon 11 using a replacement gene targeting strategy again with the vector sequences located in an adjacent intron. A significant reduction in death from intestinal blockage is observed in the G551D homozygotes compared to the survival rate of the cftr^{m1UNC} homozygotes, thus reproducing the correlation seen in humans.

Classic transgenesis

An alternative approach to gene targeting is to use pronuclear injection of fertilised mouse oocytes to introduce a CFTR cDNA transgene carrying the chosen mutation into a random site. Providing that this integration site is not on chromosome 6 (the location of the murine Cftr gene), the mice carrying the transgene can be crossed to any of the existing cystic fibrosis mutant mice. In this way the "knockout" cystic fibrosis mice can be engineered to express the ΔF508 protein. The transgene can be of either murine or, of greater interest, human origin, and tissue expression can be controlled by an appropriate choice of promoter. Lines of transgenic mice that express normal human CFTR under the control of the rat intestinal fatty-acid binding protein (FABPi)[39] have been created. The transgene directed expression of the human CFTR gene to the gut, and when the mice were crossed onto cftr^{m1UNC} animals the electrophysiological defect in the gut of the cftr^{m1UNC} animals was 30% corrected and the cystic fibrosis intestinal disease was ameliorated. Importantly functional correction was observed even though the profile of FABPi promoter driven expression was distinct from that of the endogenous murine Cftr mRNA in wild type mice.

Testing new therapeutic approaches

Before the cystic fibrosis gene was cloned, treatment was at best palliative, but now improved treatments may be developed on two complementary fronts. A molecular understanding of CFTR function will certainly aid the design of rational approaches to pharmacological intervention, and mice carrying the ΔF508 mutation may be particularly relevant. The availability of cloned CFTR expression constructs means that gene correction strategies can also be developed. Other novel treatments could be studied in appropriate animal models before clinical trials.

Somatic gene therapy

Although there is considerable understanding of CFTR function, there remains much to learn, and cloning of the gene has made possible the first steps towards gene correction treatment. If a normal copy of the CFTR gene can be introduced into affected tissues in patients with cystic fibrosis, then all of the downstream, and as yet incompletely understood consequences of CFTR gene dysfunction should be corrected. Exciting though this prospect is, it is not without its own problems. Safety of treatment assumes an overriding importance and such treatment will correct tissue damage. Ideally, such treatment must start before organs are damaged. The lung will be the first target for somatic gene treatment as this is the organ which mainly accounts for morbidity and mortality. As patients with cystic fibrosis are unpredictable in their susceptibility to infection and response to antimicrobial treatment, gene treatment will need to start in childhood. This raises important issues of informed consent and places a responsibility on scientists and physicians to ensure that the proposed method of treatment will be both safe and effective for the lifetime of the patient. Animal testing for safety is a prerequisite of any clinical trial and a preferred option must be to combine this with an assessment efficacy in a relevant animal model.

So what progress has been made down the route to gene correction treatment and where have animals, particularly the cystic fibrosis mutant mice, played a part? Before deciding on a strategy for somatic gene treatment, several competing factors must be considered and balanced. In what form is the CFTR gene to be expressed? By what route and by which cellular uptake mechanism is the transgene to be delivered? How will these choices be influenced by the desire for efficient transfer, long term stable expression, and primary safety considerations? And what of the longer term requirements, that the gene delivery system be produced to the standards required of a prescription drug? Many of these requirements are in unavoidable conflict. Application to cystic fibrosis apart, somatic gene treatment is itself a fledgling field. Treatment of cystic fibrosis by somatic gene treatment is the first proposed application in which the disease is not immediately life threatening. It is therefore unreasonable to expect that any of the currently available gene transfer systems can meet all these requirements.

Focusing specifically on the lung, the objective of therapeutic gene delivery raises both opportunities and special challenges. The lung epithelium is directly accessible and physicians and patients with cystic fibrosis are used to non-invasive aerosol drug treatments, but the purulent secretions that characterise the lung in cystic fibrosis may constitute a serious barrier to gene delivery.

Surfactant protein-C-promoter-driven expression of human CFTR in the lung and testes in transgenic mice implies that somatic gene treatment is non-toxic to the lung epithelia.[40] Once delivered, any therapeutic effect can last only for the lifetime of each terminally differentiated transfected cell. Epithelial stem cells remain elusive; experiments with xenograft rat tracheal reconstitution have suggested the rare basal cell as a candidate.[41] Efficient delivery of stable transgenes to such cells is a major challenge for the future. For the moment, full advantage must be taken of the fact that the respiratory epithelium has a slow turnover. If efficient transfer and stable expression of transgenes can be achieved, then the treatment might have to be repeated only at monthly intervals or less.

The absence of an appreciable turnover of cells rules out retroviruses for gene delivery. Attention has been concentrated on recombinant adenovirus which is naturally trophic for airways epithelial cells and which can accommodate the CFTR gene. The lung epithelium of the cotton rat was infected with CFTR recombinant adenovirus and potentially therapeutic levels of CFTR expression were obtained.[42] Based on this and additional studies in primates, several groups applied successfully to the Recombinant Advisory Committee and to the Food and Drugs Administration in the United States for permission to undertake clinical trials. Several trials are currently underway and encouraging results have been reported.[43] It is premature to comment extensively on these results and before other studies now in progress are completed, but some conclusions can be drawn. Firstly recombinant CFTR adenovirus is capable of transferring the CFTR gene and correcting the basic bioelectrical defect, but only transiently. Additionally, use of the adenovirus may elicit an inflammatory response to infection, but as bioelectrical correction was obtained at a multiplicity of infection of 1, this may be less serious than previously believed. In Rhesus monkeys and cotton rats repeated delivery of the Ad2/CFTR adenovirus is safe and efficacious.[44]

A major concern about the adenovirus vector is the stringent requirement that each batch is free of wild type virus, to remove any possibility of accidental recombination to form an infectious particle. A delivery strategy which circumvents potential problems of both adenovirus and of animal viruses is attractive. Liposomes are hypoimmunogenic, chemically defined, and can be mass produced to a defined pharmacological standard, though there is indiscriminate gene delivery and less efficient transfer than virus infection. Correction of the electrophysiological defect in cystic fibrosis mutant mice has been reported twice using CFTR cDNA transferred to the respiratory epithelium complexed with a cationic liposome.[22][45] Tracheal instillation of CFTR cDNA complexed with DOTMA/DOPE, (Lipofectin) produced complete correction of the electrophysiological defect in tracheal explants from four of six mice treated. The other two animals showed no detectable correction which was ascribed to failure of delivery.[22] In a larger study DNA was delivered by nebulisation. Using βgal as a reporter gene, the authors observed successful transfer using DOTMA/DOPE, DOTAP (also commercially available), and DC-chol/DOPE.[45] DC-chol/DOPE is approved for use in gene trials to treat melanoma and has shown no toxic effect in mice, pigs and rabbits.[46] There was no evidence of a toxic effect or histological damage in mice from DOTAP, but only DC-chol/DOPE was used to transfer the CFTR gene to the cystic fibrosis mutant mice. Partial to complete correction of the electrophysiological defect occurred in the nose (measured in vivo) and in the trachea (in vitro).

The former result is important because early clinical trials are likely to start with gene delivery to the nose where simple measurements of potential difference and drug responses can be used to measure efficacy. The latter result is equally important because it is the airway defect which must be corrected for clinical benefit. It is now important to find out how efficient, repeatable, and long lasting the effect of liposome mediated gene transfer is. On the basis of these promising results, a phase I trial involving single nasal application has been carried out in the United Kingdom (Caplan et al, unpublished observations) with reassuring toxicological data and partial electrophysiological correction.

Concluding remarks

It is clear that the cystic fibrosis mutant mice are a model for many of the hallmarks of the disease. It is likely that basic research in cystic fibrosis will benefit greatly from the null mutant mice and from the "clinically relevant" mutants. Together with the instructive species-specific differences, this promises to provide many new opportunities and stimulate novel lines of investigation. In addition to improving our understanding of the pathophysiology of the disease, these mice are certain to help speed the development of safe and effective new treatments.

Acknowledgements

JRD is supported by a Caledonian Research Fellowship, and the studies by the Medical Research Council, the Cystic Fibrosis Research Trust, and the Association Française Contre de Lutte Mucoviscidose.

This chapter is based on a previous one (Dorin JR, Alton EWFW, Porteous DJ) Mouse models for cystic fibrosis. In: Dodge J, Brock DJ, Widdicombe J, eds. *Cystic fibrosis: current topics. Vol 2.* Chichester: John Wiley, 1994.

We thank all the members of the Edinburgh Cystic Fibrosis Group for their contribution to the success of this work and Eric Alton for helpful discussions.

References

1 Snouwaert JN, Brigman KK, Latour AM *et al.* An animal model for cystic fibrosis made by gene targeting. *Science* 1992; **257**: 1083–8.

2 Dorin JR, Dickinson P, Alton EWFW *et al.* Cystic fibrosis in the mouse by targeted insertional mutagenesis. *Nature* 1992; **359**: 211–5.

3 Colledge W, Ratcliffe R, Foster D, Williamson R, Evans M. Cystic fibrosis mouse with intestinal obstruction. *Lancet* 1992; **340**: 680.

4 O'Neal WK, Hasty P, McCray PB, *et al.* A severe phenotype in mice with a duplication of exon 3 in the cystic fibrosis locus. *Hum Mol Genet* 1993; **2**: 1561–9.

5 Tata F, Stainer P, Wicking C, *et al.* Cloning the mouse homologue of the human cystic fibrosis transmembrane conductance regulator gene. *Genomics* 1991; **10**: 301–7.

6 Yorifuji T, Lemna WK, Ballard CF, *et al.* Molecular cloning and sequence analysis of the murine cDNA for the cystic fibrosis transmembrane conductance regulator gene. *Genomics* 1991; **10**: 547–50.

7 Welsh MJ. Abnormal regulation of ion channels in cystic fibrosis epithelia. *FASEB Journal* 1990; **4**: 2718–25.

8 Smith SN, Alton EWFW, Geddes DM. Ion transport characteristics of the murine trachea and caecum. *Clin Sci* 1991; **82**: 667–72.

9 Mansour SL, Thomas KR, Capecchi MR. Disruption of the proto-oncogene *int-2* in mouse embryo-derived stem cells: a general strategy for targeting mutations to non-selectable genes. *Nature* 1988; **336**: 348–53.

10 Deng C, Capecchi MR. Re-examination of gene targeting frequency as a function of the extent of homology between the targeting vector and the target locus. *Mol Cell Biol* 1992; **12**: 3365–71.

11 Moens CB, Auerbach AB, Conlan RA, Joyner AL, Rossant J. A targeted mutation reveals a role for N-Myc in branching morphogenesis in the embryonic mouse lung. *Genes and Development* 1992; **6**: 691–704.

12 Dorin JR, Stevenson BJ, Fleming S *et al.* Long term survival of the exon 10 insertional cystic fibrosis mutant mouse is a consequence of low level residual wild type Cftr gene expression. *Mammalian Genome*, in press.

13 Delaney SJ, Rich DP, Thomson SA, *et al.* Cystic Fibrosis transmembrane conductance regulator splice variants are not conserved and fail to produce chloride channels. *Nature Genetics* 1993; **4**: 426–31.

14 Chu CS, Trapnell B, Murtagh J, *et al.* Variable deletion of exon 9 coding sequences in cystic fibrosis transmembrane conductance regulator gene mRNA transcripts in normal bronchial epithelium. *EMBO J* 1991; **10**: 1355–63.

15 Clarke LL, Grubb BR, Gabriel SE, *et al.* Defective epithelial chloride transport in a gene-targeted mouse model of cystic fibrosis. *Science* 1992; **257**: 1125–8.

16 Ratcliff R, Evans MJ, Cuthbert AW, *et al.* Production of a severe cystic fibrosis mutation in mice by gene targeting. *Nature Genetics* 1992; **4**: 35–41.

17 Dorin J, Alton EWFW, Porteous DJ. Mouse models for cystic fibrosis. In: *Cystic fibrosis: current topics. Vol 2.* Dodge JA, Brock DJH, Widdicombe JH, eds. Chichester: John Wiley; 1994.

18 Clarke LL, Grubb BR, Yankaskas JR, Cotton CU, McKenzie A, Boucher RC. Relationship of a non-cystic fibrosis transmembrane conductance regulator-mediated chloride conductance to organ level disease in Cftr (-/-) mice. *Proc Nat Acad Sci USA* 1994; **91**: 479–83.

19 Gray MA, Winpenny JP, Porteous DJ, Dorin JR, Argent BE. CFTR and calcium-activated chloride currents in pancreatic duct cells of a transgenic CF mouse. *Am J Physiol* 1994: C213–C221.

20 Hyde S, Gill D, Higgins C, *et al.* Correction of the ion transport defect in cystic fibrosis transgenic mice by gene therapy. *Nature* 1993; **362**: 250–5.

21 Knowles M, Gatzy J, Boucher RC. Increased bioelectric potential difference across respiratory epithelia in cystic fibrosis. *N Engl J Med* 1981; **305**: 1489–95.

22 Alton EWFW, Currie D, Logan-Sinclair R, *et al.* Nasal potential difference: a clinical diagnostic test for cystic fibrosis. *Eur Resp J* 1990; **3**: 922–6.

23 Englehardt JF, Yankaskas JR, Ernst SA, *et al.* Submucosal glands are the predominant site of CFTR expression in human bronchus. *Nature Genetics* 1992; **2**: 240–8.

24 Boat T, Welsh MJ, Beaudet A. Cystic fibrosis. In: Scriver CL, Beaudet AL, Sly WS, Valle D, eds. *The metabolic basis of inherited disease.* New York: McGraw Hill; 1989: 2649–80.

25 Trezise AEO, Buchwald M. In vivo cell-specific expression of the cystic fibrosis transmembrane conductance regulator. *Nature* 1991; **353**: 434–7.

26 Engelhardt JF, Zepeda M, Cohn JA, Yankaskas JR, Wilson JM. *J Clin Invest* 1994; **93**: 737–49.

27 Yoshimura K, Nakamura H, Trapnell BC, *et al.* Expression of the cystic fibrosis transmembrane conductance regulator gene in cells of non-epithelial origin. *Nucl Acids Res* 1991; **19**: 5417–23.

28 Porteous DJ, Dorin JR. How relevant are mouse models for human diseases to somatic gene therapy? *Tibtech* 1993; **11**: 173–81.

29 The cystic fibrosis genotype-phenotype consortium. Correlation between genotype and phenotype in patients with cystic fibrosis. *N Engl J Med* 1993; **329**: 1308–12.

30 Kubesch P, Dork T, Wullbrand U, *et al.* Genetic determinants of airways' colonisation with Pseudomonas aeruginosa in cystic fibrosis. *Lancet* 1993; **341**: 189–93.

31 Sheppard DN, Rich DP, Ostedgaard LS, *et al.* Mutations in CFTR associated with mild-disease-form CI channels with altered pore properties. *Nature* 1993; **362**: 160–4.

32 Colledge WH, Abella BS, Southern KW *et al.* Generation and characterization of a ΔF508 cystic fibrosis mouse model. *Nature Genetics* 1994; **10**: 445–50.

33 van Doorninck JH, French PJ, Verbeek E *et al.* A mouse model for the cystic fibrosis ΔF508 mutation. *EMBO J* 1995; **14**: 4403–11.

34 Hasty P, Ramirez-Solls R, Krumlauf R, Bradley A. Introduction of a subtle mutation into the Hox-2.6 locus in embryonic stem cells. *Nature* 1991; **350**: 243–6.

35 Valancius V, Smithies O. Testing an "in-out" targeting procedure for making subtle genomic modifications in mouse embryonic stem cells. *Mol Cell Biol* 1991; **11**: 1402–8.

36 Deng C, Thomas KR, Capecchi MR. Location of crossovers during gene targeting with insertion and replacement vectors. *Mol Cell Biol* 1993; **13**: 2134–40.

37 Delaney SJ, Alton EWFW, Smith S, *et al.* A cystic fibrosis mouse model carrying

the common human missense mutation G5551D. *EMBO J*, in press.

38 Hamosh A, King TM, Rosenstein BJ, *et al.* Cystic fibrosis patients bearing both the common missense mutations gly-asp at codon 551 and the Δ508 mutation are clinically indistinguishable from ΔF508 homozygotes except for decreased risk of meconium ileus. *Am J Hum Genet* 1992.

39 Zhou L, Dey CR, Wert SE, DuVall MD, Frizzell RA, Whitsett JA. Correction of lethal intestinal defect in a mouse model of cystic fibrosis by human CFTR. *Science* 1994; **266**: 1705–8.

40 Whitsett JA, Dey CR, Stripp BR, *et al.* Human cystic fibrosis transmembrane conductance regulator directed to respiratory epithelial cells of transgenic mice. *Nature Genetics* 1992; **2**: 13–20.

41 Englehardt JF, Yang Y, Stratford-Perricaudet LD, *et al.* Direct gene transfer of human CFTR into human bronchial epithelia of zenografts with E1-deleted adenoviruses. *Nature Genetics* 1993; **4**: 27–34.

42 Rosenfeld MA, Yoshimura K, Trapnell BC, *et al.* In vivo transfer of the human cystic fibrosis transmembrane conductance regulator gene to the airway epithelium. *Cell* 1992; **68**: 143–55.

43 Zabner J, Couture LA, Gregory RJ, *et al.* Adenovirus-mediated gene transfer transiently corrects the chloride transport defect in nasal epithelia of patients with cystic fibrosis. *Cell* 1993; **75**: 207–16.

44 Zabner J, Petersen DM, Puga AP, *et al.* Safety and efficacy of repetitive adenovirus mediated transfer of cDNA to airway epithelia of primates and cotton rats. *Nature Genetics* 1994; **6**: 75–83.

45 Alton EWFW, Middleton PG, Caplen NJ, *et al.* Non-invasive liposome-mediated gene delivery can correct the ion transport defect in cystic fibrosis mutant mice. *Nature Genetics* 1993; **5**: 135–42.

46 Stewart MJ, Plautz GE, del Buono L, *et al.* Gene transfer *in vivo* with DNA-liposome complexes: safety and acute toxicity in mice. *Hum Gene Therap* 1992; **3**: 267–75.

4 The cystic fibrosis gene

ALAN W CUTHBERT

Cystic fibrosis is an autosomal recessive disease characterised by thick viscid secretions in the airways and intestines (often blocking the lumen in the latter), excessive salt secretion in the sweat, pancreatic insufficiency caused by the blockage of the pancreatic duct with mucus, male infertility, and sometimes liver failure. Opportunistic infections of the airways are responsible for a great deal of the morbidity and mortality, the mucus filled airways providing a rich environment for organisms, such as *Pseudomonas* species (Chapter 6). By contrast, the cystic fibrosis heterozygote is normal, and heterozygosity may confer a genetic advantage. Because heterozygotes contain both the normal and the mutant allele, the presence of the mutation does not interfere with the production or function of the normal gene product. If the genetic sequence for the normal gene product can be introduced into somatic cells of patients with cystic fibrosis therefore, it is expected that generation of the normal gene product will lead to normal function and hence a treatment for the disease. Furthermore, if the gene product was stably expressed throughout the lifetime of the cells then treatment might be required only at infrequent intervals. Even more attractive is the possibility that normal gene expression could be introduced into stem cells, resulting in the permanent expression of the gene product in diseased cells and a permanent cure for the disease. Augmentation of the genetic information in somatic cells is called gene therapy, and currently considered to be a major hope for patients with the disease.

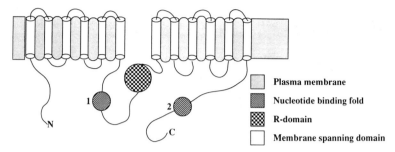

Figure 4.1   A proposed structure for the cystic fibrosis transmembrane conductance regulator embedded in the lipid bilayer of the cell membrane.

The cystic fibrosis gene product

All the possibilities alluded to above are a consequence of the discovery of the cystic fibrosis gene in 1989.[1-3] Since then the functional responsibilities of the gene product have become clearer and much of this review is concerned with this. There is no doubt that cystic fibrosis is an epithelial disease, but whether correction of the transporting characteristics of the epithelial cells themselves will correct all the features of the disease such as abnormal mucus production and the susceptibility to bacterial infections is as yet not clear.

The cystic fibrosis gene codes for a 1480 amino acid protein called the cystic fibrosis transmembrane conductance regulator (CFTR). The gene is large and consists of a quarter of a million bases with 24 exons. In the most common cystic fibrosis mutation a single codon, that for phenylalanine at position 508, is missing, so a defective protein, ΔF508 CFTR, is produced. This mutation accounts for 70% of those detected in patients with cystic fibrosis in the United Kingdom. More than 400 mutations in the cystic fibrosis gene have now been described, however, and there is a considerable interest in relating phenotype to genotype. For example, in general patients with cystic fibrosis who are homozygous for ΔF508 have both severe pulmonary symptoms and pancreatic insufficiency.

Figure 4.1 shows a diagram of CFTR. While this gives an idea of the probable arrangement of the constituent parts it is not an architectural plan of the CFTR molecule. The molecule consists of symmetrical halves joined at the R-domain. Each half has six membrane spanning domains and a nucleotide binding fold which binds ATP. Phenylalanine 508 is located in the nucleotide binding

53

fold nearest to the N-terminus. The R-domain contains many sites for phosphorylation by protein kinases A and C. The epithelial tissues that are affected in cystic fibrosis are either anion secreting (pancreatic duct, epididymus), cation absorbing (sweat gland duct), or both (airways). Generally the secreted anion is chloride, but it may be bicarbonate as in the pancreatic duct and gall bladder. In the absorptive sweat gland sodium ions are absorbed together with chloride as a counter-ion. The main biophysical lesion in cystic fibrosis is the inability of agents which raise cyclic adenosine monophosphate (cAMP) within cells to increase the chloride conductance, so preventing chloride secretion or, in the case of the sweat glands, preventing cation absorption because of the inability of the accompanying chloride to be absorbed as well.

It has become clear that the protein coded for by the cystic fibrosis gene is an epithelial cell membrane chloride channel — that is, CFTR is a chloride channel which is sensitive to cAMP, the channel opening as a result of phosphorylation. The assumption is that protein kinase A is activated by cAMP, which in the presence of ATP phosphorylates the channel. Some of the evidence by which this is based is given below.

CFTR as a chloride channel

CFTR has been shown by immunostaining to be present in the apical membranes of pancreatic duct cells, salivary gland ducts, crypt cells of the large and small intestine, and cells lining the airways.[4-6] Human fetal lung shows a decreasing gradient of CFTR mRNA from the proximal to the distal pulmonary epithelium[7] so CFTR and its messenger RNA occur at sites which are expected if indeed the protein acts as an epithelial chloride channel. Particularly important is the apical location of the staining because well acknowledged models of chloride secretion require that location for chloride channels.

Transfection of cells in culture is easily achieved using either viral vectors in which the CFTR sequence is incorporated or by the calcium phosphate precipitation method. Transfecting cystic fibrosis cells in culture with the CFTR sequence conferred a cAMP sensitive chloride conductance on the cells, a phenomenon that did not occur when the ΔF508 CFTR sequence was used.[8 9] Furthermore, cells that do not normally express CFTR, for example HeLa cells, show a cAMP sensitive chloride conductance after transfection with the CFTR sequence.[10 11]

Transfection of HeLa cells with the sequence for CFTR gave a cAMP sensitive anion conductance with a permeability sequence bromide > chloride > iodide > fluoride. Site-directed mutagenesis was then employed to modify the sequence so that when translated the basic amino acids lysine 95 and lysine 335 were converted to aspartate and glutamate, respectively. Transfection with the modified sequence gave anion selectivity with the order iodide > bromide > chloride > fluoride.[12] In other words modification of the amino acid sequence in CFTR changed the anion selectivity of the ion channel. Both the modified residues lie at the outer end of two of the membrane-spanning segments. The membrane-spanning domains are thought to arrange themselves within the membrane to form a channel for ion permeation, so it is perhaps not surprising that modification of the charge around the end of the channel leads to a change in ion selectivity. It has also been suggested that blocking and unblocking of the channel results from the movement of the R-domain into and out of the membrane pore, a mechanism previously proposed for potassium channels.

Transfection of cells with ΔR CFTR sequence (with coding for the R-domain removed) conferred a chloride conductance on HeLa cells which did not require cAMP for activation, suggesting that in the absence of the R-domain the channel cannot close.[13]

Recombinant CFTR protein was incorporated into lipid bilayers and conferred anion channel activity when protein kinase A and ATP were added.[14] As the experimental system in this instance consisted of only purified CFTR and lipids it is difficult to escape the conclusion that CFTR is a chloride channel. With symmetrical bathing solutions on either side of the membrane the CFTR chloride channel has a conductance of 10–20 pS, a linear current voltage relationship, with a selectivity sequence of nitrate > chloride > bicarbonate, and impermeable to anions such as gluconate.

Intracellular protein trafficking

Despite this strong evidence that CFTR functions as an epithelial chloride channel there are observations that modify this simple view that CFTR forms a functional channel while the mutant form, ΔF508 CFTR, cannot do so.

When the ΔF508 sequence was introduced into *Xenopus* oocytes or Vero cells a cAMP-dependent chloride conductance appeared, though its development was slower and the extent less than with the native protein.[15,16]

55

Expression of ΔF508 CFTR in 3T3 fibroblasts at 37°C did not confer a chloride conductance as expected, but after incubation at 30°C for 24 hours a cAMP sensitive anion conductance developed.[17] This finding is consistent with those in the previous paragraph, as oocytes were also cultured at a low temperature.

The findings given in the two previous paragraphs are difficult to understand until one considers the localisation of CFTR. CFTR is a glycosylated membrane protein of 165 kDa, while the non-glycosylated form is only 145 kDa. Cells transfected with ΔF508 CFTR produce little glycosylated protein. It was proposed that the mutant protein failed to be processed and transported properly within the cell and was not inserted into the cell membrane.[18 19] Further, ΔF508 CFTR was improperly localised in human cystic fibrosis sweat glands.[4] It seems that in cystic fibrosis there is altered intracellular CFTR protein trafficking which can be alleviated in vitro by reducing temperature. If the mutant protein does not reach the membrane it shows chloride channel activity. These findings raise the possibility that if the intracellular protein trafficking processes become amenable to pharmacological manipulation the delivery of the mutant protein to the membrane may be increased, with a consequent improvement in function. However, this implies that the quality control mechanisms in the cell are suppressed, which may have other consequences for cellular function.

Other mutations

In the United Kingdom the ΔF508 variation accounts for 70% of mutations in the cystic fibrosis gene while in the Mediterranean area this figure is about 50%, but there are 400 other mutations described in the cystic fibrosis gene. With the ΔF508 mutation there is a failure of translation processing as with a number of other mutations, but nonsense, frameshift, and splice mutations are also known and in general give either no protein or truncated proteins that are rapidly degraded; hence no functional activity can exist in these circumstances. Other rare mutations exist in which the regulation of the CFTR protein by ATP is deficient and yet others which affect the membrane spanning domains leading to chloride channels with low conductance.[20]

There is intense interest in the relation between genotype and phenotype but this is not yet sufficiently understood to be useful in formulating treatment or predicting the course of the disease. For example, the ΔF508 homozygote has a high sweat chloride, severe pulmonary disease, and pancreatic insufficiency.[21] By contrast, heterozygotes with ΔF508/F508C (cysteine substituting for phenylalanine at position 508) have no pulmonary disease, normal pancreatic function, and normal sweat chloride. Such people are no different from carriers, but produce no wild type protein.[22] Presumably F508C is a CFTR analogue which is transported to the membrane and functions equivalently to the native protein. An even more surprising example is ΔF508/R117H (arginine replaced with histidine at position 117) which in men leads to a congenital absence of the vas deferens and no other symptoms.[23] It is possible that mutations will be discovered in which chloride channel activity is increased, perhaps with permanent secretory diarrhoea as a phenotype. Such mutations might be useful in some forms of gene treatment where delivery can be achieved only with low efficiency.

Animal models of cystic fibrosis

The lack of a satisfactory animal model for cystic fibrosis has hindered research which until recently depended on tissues or cell lines derived from patients with cystic fibrosis. Three laboratories described the creation of cystic fibrosis mice almost simultaneously using essentially the same strategy (chapter 3).[24-26]

Epithelial tissues from these mice showed the cystic fibrosis phenotype with epithelium lining the trachea, colon and caecum failing to show cAMP-dependent chloride secretion.[25 27 28] There are two accounts of attempts to reverse the cystic fibrosis of phenotype in mice by gene therapy. In one study the Cftr sequence was incorporated into a plasmid pREP8 and formulated in a liposome vector, which was then instilled into the tracheas of cystic fibrosis mice.[29] Control mice were either cystic fibrosis mice or normal mice given plasmid without the Cftr sequence. After two days the animals were killed and the tracheal and caecal epithelia examined for their phenotypes in a blind study. In the cystic fibrosis mice given the Cftr sequence the phenotype of the intestinal epithelium was unchanged while that of the trachea was normal. In a similar study using a different line of cystic fibrosis mice in which a mixture of three different plasmids containing the Cftr sequence was given by nebulisation in a liposome vector the phenotype of the tracheal epithelium was again changed towards normality; in particular, the cAMP-dependent chloride secretion was increased.[30] In both studies, however, there were important differences in the biophysical characteristics of the tracheal epithelium compared with those reported in humans. For example, the amiloride sensitive current was less in the cystic fibrosis tissues than in normal or treated cystic fibrosis tissues, while it may have been expected that the epithelium would be hyperabsorbing as in humans. Furthermore, in intact tracheal epithelium from cystic fibrosis mice there was a small response to forskolin (which leads to cAMP accumulation) which was not present in cultured murine cystic fibrosis tracheal epithelium.[28] Nevertheless, while these differences require further investigation the reversal of the phenotype indicates the usefulness of the animal model for investigating genetic strategies for treatment. Recently a ΔF508 mouse model was described.[31] Epithelia from the airways and alimentary canal are phenotypically cystic fibrosis like. Airway cells cultured at 27°C developed a cAMP-dependent chloride conductance, indicating the ΔF508 protein is produced, but normally does not reach its correct location in the cell. This animal model will be useful for investigating procedures which overcome the trafficking defect for ΔF508 Cftr. If normalisation of phenotype can be achieved with pharmacological agents an alternative to gene therapy for cystic fibrosis will have been achieved.

It is not yet clear what will be the best vehicle for gene therapy in humans and a great deal of effort is currently being put into adenoviral vectors. Adenoviruses commonly infect the airways and the gastrointestinal tract and their tropism for these sites conveys an advantage compared with non-specific vectors, such as liposomes. In recombinant vectors part of the viral genome is replaced by the CFTR sequence so that they can enter the target cell but express only the recombinant gene. There is some concern, however, that repeated exposure may lead to immunological responses. It is also possible that these disabled viruses could replicate with help from coincident adenovirus infection.

Finally, lung epithelial cells have a long lifetime, probably about 40 days. Transfection of airway epithelial cells with stable expression of CFTR for the lifetime of the cell might mean that monthly treatment would be sufficient, but eventually the treatment of dysfunction in the alimentary tract, pancreas, liver, and biliary tree will need to be studied. These will present different problems, particularly as intestinal epithelial cells have a lifetime of only a few days. It will then be necessary to target stem cells, perhaps using retroviral vectors which integrate into the genome, but with some risk of insertional mutagenesis. Interested readers may wish to consult a recent review.[32] Experimental attempts have been made to transfect cells with retroviral vectors ex vivo and then to seed these in vivo. Rat bronchial epithelial cells, after transfections, were xenografted on to denuded rat tracheas which were then implanted into nu/nu mice.[33] Using a reporter gene it was shown that a fully differentiated epithelium that expressed the reporter spread across the graft, showing that stem cells had been successfully transfected. Whether such an ex vivo approach will ever be useful in the treatment of human cystic fibrosis currently seems doubtful.

Preliminary clinical trials

In several clinical trials attempts have been made to normalise the electrophysiological characteristics of the nasal epithelium in cystic fibrosis patients. In two an adenoviral vector was used, and in another liposome mediated gene transfer was employed.[34–36] Thus far the results are disappointing with only modest or no change in characteristics. It appears that the fraction of epithelial cells transfected is very small and there is an urgent need to find ways to increase the efficiency of gene transfer.

References

1 Rommens JM, Iannuzzi MC, Kerem B, et al. Identification of the cystic fibrosis gene: chromosomal walking and jumping. Science 1989; 243: 1059–65.

2 Riordan JR, Rommens JM, Kerem B, et al. Identification of the cystic fibrosis gene: cloning and characterisation of the complementary DNA. Science 1989; 245: 1066–72.

3 Kerem B, Rommens JM, Buchanan JA, et al. Identification of the cystic fibrosis gene: genetic analysis. Science 1989; 245: 1073–80.

4 Kartner N, Augustina O, Jensen TJ, et al. Mislocalisation of ΔF508 CFTR in cystic fibrosis sweat gland. Nature Genetics 1992; 1: 321–7.

5 Marino CR, Matovcik LM, Gorelick FS et al. Localisation of the cystic fibrosis transmembrane conductance regulator in pancreas. J Clin Invest 1991; 88: 712–6.

6 Rosenfeld MA, Yoshimura K, Trapnell BC, et al. In vivo transfer of the human cystic fibrosis transmembrane conductance regulator gene to the airway epithelium. Cell 1992; 68: 143–55.

7 McCray PB, Wohlford-Lenane CL, Snyder JM. Localisation of cystic fibrosis transmembrane conductance regulator mRNA in human fetal lung tissue by in situ hybridization. J Clin Invest 1992; 90: 619–25.

8 Gregory RJ, Cheng SH, Rich DP, et al. Expression and characterisation of the cystic fibrosis transmembrane conductance regulator. Nature 1990; 347: 382–6.

9 Rich DP, Anderson MP, Gregory RJ, et al. Expression of cystic fibrosis transmembrane conductance regulator corrects defective chloride channel regulation in cystic fibrosis airway epithelial cells. Nature 1990; 347: 358–63.

10 Rommens JM, Dho S, Bear CE, et al. cAMP-inducible chloride conductance in mouse fibroblast lines stably expressing the human cystic fibrosis transmembrane conductance regulator. Proc Natl Acad Sci USA 1991; 88: 7500–4.

11 Anderson MP, Rich DP, Gregory RJ, et al. Generation of cAMP-activated chloride currents by expression of CFTR. Science 1991; 251: 679–82.

12 Anderson MP, Gregory RJ, Thompson S, et al. Demonstration that CFTR is a chloride channel by alteration of its anion selectivity. *Science* 1991; **253**: 202–5.

13 Rich DP, Gregory RJ, Anderson MP, et al. Effect of deleting the R-domain on CFTR-generated chloride channels. *Science* 1991; **253**: 205–7.

14 Bear CE, Li C, Kartner N, et al. Purification and functional reconstitution of the cystic fibrosis transmembrane conductance regulator (CFTR). *Cell* 1992; **66**: 809–18.

15 Drumm ML, Wilkinson DJ, Smith LS, et al. Chloride conductance expressed by ΔF508 and other mutant CFTRs in *Xenopus* oocytes. *Science* 1991; **254**: 1797–9.

16 Dalesmans W, Babry P, Champigny G, et al. Altered chloride ion channel kinetics associated with the ΔF508 cystic fibrosis mutation. *Nature* 1991; **354**: 526–8.

17 Denning GM, Anderson MP, Amara AF, et al. Processing of mutant cystic fibrosis transmembrane conductance regulator is temperature-sensitive. *Nature* 1992; **358**: 761–4.

18 Cheng SH, Gregory RJ, Marshall J, et al. Defective intracellular transport and processing of CFTR is the molecular basis of most cystic fibrosis. *Cell* 1990; **63**: 827–34.

19 Zeitlin PL, Crawford I, Lu L, et al. CFTR protein expression in primary and cultured epithelia. *Proc Natl Acad Sci USA* 1992; **89**: 344–7.

20 Welsh MJ, Smith AE. Molecular mechanisms of CFTR chloride channel dysfunction in cystic fibrosis. *Cell* 1993; **73**: 1251–4.

21 Kerem E, Corey M, Kerem B-S, et al. The relation between genotype and phenotype in cystic fibrosis-analysis of the most common mutation (delta F508) *N Engl J Med* 1991; **323**: 1517–22.

22 Kobayashi K, Knowles MR, Boucher RC, et al. Benign missense variations of the cystic fibrosis gene. *Am J Hum Genet* 1990; **47**: 611–5.

23 Anguiano A, Oates R, Amos J, et al. Congenital bilateral absence of the vas deferens: a primarily genital form of cystic fibrosis. *JAMA* 1992; **267**: 1794–7.

24 Colledge WH, Ratcliff R, Foster D, et al. Cystic fibrosis mouse with intestinal obstruction. *Lancet* 1992; **340**: 680.

25 Dorin JR, Dickinson P, Alton EWFW, et al. Cystic fibrosis in the mouse by targeted insertional mutation. *Nature* 1992; **359**: 211–5.

26 Snouwaert JN, Brigman KK, Latour AM, et al. An animal model for cystic fibrosis made by gene targeting. *Science* 1992; **257**: 1083–8.

27 Ratcliff R, Evans MJ, Cuthbert AW, et al. Production of a severe cystic fibrosis mutation in mice. *Nature Genetics* 1993; **4**: 35–41.

28 Clarke LL, Grubb BR, Gabriel SE, et al. Defective epithelial chloride transport in a gene targetted mouse model of cystic fibrosis. *Science* 1992; **257**: 1125–8.

29 Hyde SC, Gill DR, Higgins CF, et al. Correction of the ion channel defect in cystic fibrosis transgenic mice by gene therapy. *Nature* 1993; **362**: 250–5.

30 Alton EWFW, Middleton PG, Caplen NJ, et al. Non-invasive liposome-mediated gene delivery can correct the ion transport defect in cystic fibrosis mutant mice. *Nature Genetics* 1993; **5**: 135–42.

31 Colledge WH, Abella BS, Southern KW, et al. Generation and characterisation of a ΔF508 cystic fibrosis mouse model. *Nature Genetics* 1995; **10**: 445–52.

32 Flotte TR. Prospects for virus based gene therapy for cystic fibrosis. *J Bioenerg Biomembr* 1993; **25**: 37–42.

33 Engelhardt JF, Allen ED, Wilson JM. Reconstitution of tracheal grafts with a genetically modified epithelium. *Proc Natl Acad Sci USA* 1991; **88**: 1192–96.

34 Knowles MR, Hohneker KW, Zhou Z, et al. A controlled study of adenoviral-vector-mediated gene transfer in the nasal epithelium of patients with cystic fibrosis. *N Engl J Med* 1995; **333**: 823–31.

35 Caplen NJ, Alton EWFW, Middleton PG, et al. Liposome-mediated CFTR gene transfer to the nasal epithelium of patients with cystic fibrosis. *Nature*

Medicine 1995; **1**: 39–46.

36 Zabner J, Couture LA, Gregory RJ, Graham SM, Smith AE, Welsh MJ. Adenovirus-mediated gene transfer transiently corrects the chloride transplant defect in nasal epithelia of patients with cystic fibrosis. *Cell* 1993; **75**: 207–10.

5 Lung injury

DENNIS SHALE, J S ELBORN

As the life span of patients with cystic fibrosis increases, the major cause of death in adults is respiratory failure associated with pulmonary hypertension and cor pulmonale.[1] A variable period of chronic pulmonary infection and progressive lung injury precedes this and is associated with considerable morbidity in older children and adult patients. A continuous and exuberant host inflammatory response to the presence of chronic endobronchial bacterial infection is the main cause of lung injury. The initiation of the infective process, the regulation of the inflammatory response, and the consequences of such processes are becoming understood and may indicate ways of protecting the lungs and prolonging survival.

Pathology of the lung in cystic fibrosis

Histological abnormalities in the airways are evident within the first few days of life.[2] Submucosal gland hypertrophy, duct obstruction, and mucus cell hyperplasia occur before any confirmed infective episodes; these changes in secretion are probably related to the underlying genetic defect and lead to viscous secretions, airway casts and obstruction, which may enhance colonisation of the respiratory tract by micro-organisms. Repeated pulmonary infection, particularly viral infection, during the first year of life may add to the problem of airways obstruction by inducing a bronchiolar inflammatory response (Figure 5.1). This combination of infection and obstruction may be the nidus which allows bacterial infection, and leads to further bronchiolitis, mucus impaction, cyst formation, and ultimately bronchiectasis, which has been observed in children as young as 2 months of age.[3] Once initiated, there is a vicious cycle of endobronchial and endobronchiolar infection and inflammation with further impaired ciliary function and reduced airways clearance (Figure 5.1).[4-6]

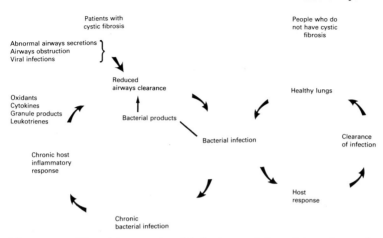

Figure 5.1 The vicious cycle of infection and lung injury in cystic fibrosis. The interaction between recurrent bacterial infection and abnormalities of airways clearance are emphasised in the formation of a vicious cycle of injury and infection in cystic fibrosis in comparison with the normal host inflammatory response and clearance that occurs in people who do not have cystic fibrosis.

Further bronchial and bronchiolar wall damage develops leading to obstruction, bronchial compression, and secondary alveolar injury with atelectasis.[6]

The role of infection

Viruses

Viral infections may directly reduce the defences of the airways and encourage secondary bacterial infection of the lower airways. It is potentially important that the major viral infections that affect the airways during the first few years of life cause bronchiolitis; that is the same portion of the airways attacked by bacterial infection in cystic fibrosis. Infection with the respiratory syncytial virus may be a factor in the acquisition of *Pseudomonas aeruginosa* infection.[7-12] Viral infections not only increase the chance of acquiring bacterial infection but also influence the state of chronic colonisation.[12] Of 300 patients reviewed at the Danish cystic fibrosis centre, two thirds first had *Ps aeruginosa* isolated from their sputum in the period October to March, and 70% started their chronic colonisation in the same winter months, the peak period for viral infections in Denmark.

Of equal importance is the role of super-added viral infection in

63

Main bacteria that affect the lungs in cystic fibrosis

- *Staph aureus*
- *H influenzae*
- *Pseudomonads*
- *Burkholderia cepacia*

---

patients with chronic bronchial infection. Respiratory symptoms may be exacerbated by such viral infections in 17%–39% of episodes.[7-11] Indeed, influenza infection may have severe consequences in adult patients, which makes immunisation each autumn worthwhile.[10] There is no evidence, however, that viral infections are more common in patients with cystic fibrosis, but they do have more impact on patients with pre-existing abnormalities of the airways.

Bacteria

The main bacteria that affect the lungs are *Staphylococcus aureus*, *Haemophilus influenzae*, and *Ps aeruginosa*. Others include a range of pseudomonads (*Ps maltophilia, Ps stutzeri* and *Ps fluoresens)* and *Burkholderia cepacia,* formerly known as *Ps cepacia*.[13] The relationship between the presence of an organism in the sputum and lung injury is not clear, which has led to the use of the term "colonisation" to indicate a non-injurious infected state and "infection" to indicate injury associated with the presence of bacteria. The use of the term "colonisation" without proof of the absence of lung injury has led clinicians to underestimate the potential for early lung injury. This is further complicated by the known low virulence that these bacteria exhibit in patients who do not have cystic fibrosis and who have intact clearance mechanisms and structurally normal airways. The first culture of *Ps aeruginosa* in adults, however, was associated with increases in circulating surrogate markers of the pulmonary inflammatory response to concentrations seen in patients with chronic colonisation (C-reactive protein (CRP), and neutrophil elastase-α_1-antiproteinase complex).[14]

Staph aureus

Staph aureus is associated with infection in the first few years of life, but there remains controversy about the importance of such infection as an initiator of lung injury. Deterioration of lung function with chronic *Staph aureus* infection before colonisation with *Ps aeruginosa* indicates this organism's capacity to initiate lung injury,[15] as does radiographic evidence of lung destruction associated with high titres of IgG antibodies to staphylococcal teichoic acid.[16] The lack of consensus about the role of *Staph aureus* has led to a diversity of treatment regimens ranging from no treatment to intermittent intensive courses aimed at eradication and continuous long term prophylaxis.[17-19] Chronic *Staph aureus* infection usually precedes *Ps aeruginosa* infection, but how such infection or its treatment relates to chronic infection with *Ps aeruginosa* is not clear.[19]

H influenzae

Non-capsulate strains of *H influenzae* are often isolated from the respiratory tract of children with cystic fibrosis though there remains debate about their role as pathogens.[20 21] Non-capsulate strains are an important pathogen in the respiratory tract in adults and in children with otitis media and community-acquired pneumonia.[22,23] *H influenzae* has increased mucosal adherence during viral infection and produces a range of virulence factors which lyse IgA_1, cause ciliary dyskinesia, release histamine, and stimulate mucus secretion.[24-26] Patients with cystic fibrosis have a higher rate of isolation of *H influenzae* than control asthmatic patients with a further increase during symptomatic respiratory deterioration.[27] In adults the role of *H influenzae* infection is probably underestimated as it may coexist with *Ps aeruginosa* in a spheroplastic form and cannot be isolated without the use of selective media.[28] When sought in the sputum of patients with cystic fibrosis infected with *Ps aeruginosa* there was 80% coinfection with *H influenzae*.[29]

Ps aeruginosa

Great interest has focused on the role of *Ps aeruginosa* in chronic infection which is associated with chronic lung injury and reduced survival.[30 31] Much of our knowledge of the host response in cystic fibrosis and its relation to lung injury comes from the study of the interaction between the host and *Ps aeruginosa* (see Chapter 6).

The effects of *Ps aeruginosa* exoproducts on cytokine mediators

Exoproducts produced by *Ps aeruginosa* may directly influence the inflammatory response of the host in favour of the bacterium.

Both elastase and alkaline protease may affect the bioactivity of interleukin 2 (IL-2), γ-interferon (IFNγ) and tumour necrosis factor-α (TNFα). Most data comes from *in vitro* studies and *in vivo* effects are largely unknown. Though the potential for such effects remains to be disproved they are unlikely to be important because most are antiinflammatory and inhibit cytokine activity, while there is no evidence of a reduced inflammatory response in patients.

Interleukin-2 (IL-2), a T-cell growth factor, is inactivated by elastase and alkaline protease[32] and the pigment pyocyanin inhibits IL-2 production and the expression of its receptor by T-cells.[33 34] So there is the potential for inhibition of T-cell-mediated antigen-specific immunity.[35] The function of IFNγ may be impaired by proteolytic enzymes,[35-38] leading to reduced T-cell function and, with the down-regulation of other pre-T-cell cytokines, a possible reduction in the immune response.[39]

Of greater importance is the potential disruption of cytokine networks, such as that regulating infiltration of the lung by neutrophils, and their activation during passage from the circulation to the air space.[38] TNFα, secreted by alveolar and airways macrophages, is likely to be a major direct activator of neutrophils in the vicinity of the airways and, secondarily, as a costimulator with IL-1β of the production and release of IL-8 by lung epithelial type II cells and fibroblasts.[40] The potential disruption of this pathway, leading to a deranged network of cytokine activity, has been suggested by various in vitro studies, but has not been shown to be active in vivo.

It is likely that the major factor governing the colonisation of the lungs with *Ps aeruginosa* is abnormal structure of the airways leading to reduced clearance mechanisms. Virulence factors are probably most important at the time of acquisition when they may increase bacterial retention in the airways.

Potential effects of *Ps aeruginosa* products on cytokine function

- Elastase and alkaline protease inactivate IL-2
- IFNγ function impaired by proteolytic enzymes
- Pyocyanin inhibits IL-2 production
- TNFα activation of neutrophils impaired
- TNFα and IL-1β stimulation of the production and release of IL-8 impaired

---

The host response to pulmonary infection

There is no convincing evidence to suggest a defect in host defences, though there are reports of individual abnormalities. Infection at sites other than the lung are no more common in patients with cystic fibrosis than in people without cystic fibrosis, and the systemic spread of pulmonary infection apart from *B cepacia* is extremely rare, despite the enormous bacterial load and often debilitated state of patients with cystic fibrosis. It is likely that the host response is largely responsible for lung injury secondary to an unremitting immunoinflammatory response to infection. Various host cells and mediators are likely to be involved in the injury process, though there are considerable gaps in our knowledge about the inter-relationship.

Pulmonary macrophages

The subpopulations of the pulmonary macrophage comprise the alveolar/airways macrophage, the interstitial macrophage, and the intravascular pulmonary macrophage.[41] The role of these subtypes in the pathogenesis of lung disease is not clear, but pulmonary macrophages with their range of functions are likely to be fundamental to the initiation and maintenance of the host response to infection (Figure 5.2). The airways and mucosal macrophages are probably the first line of defence that is met by invading bacteria. Phagocytosis will activate the cell, leading to a range of signals that affect the function of other inflammatory cells.[42] Such signals include surface membrane expression or secretion, or both, of various cytokines (for example, IL-1β, TNFα, IL-6, and IL-8), HLA class I and II antigens and the presentation of processed antigens. By this means the acute inflammatory/phagocytic response mediated by neutrophils, monocytes, and the inflammatory immune response mediated by lymphocytes, are activated and maintained. All these functions are essentially protective, and with its stimulatory effects on fibroblast proliferation and the secretion of connective tissue proteins, the pulmonary macrophage links the normally self-limiting inflammatory response to the first phases of healing. In cystic fibrosis, however, this host-protective process is maintained and exaggerated by the continual presence of bacteria and possibly by their antigenically active byproducts. This perpetuates the vicious cycle, and more tissue injury leads to more infection and further inflammation.[4]

The alveolar macrophage has a limited capacity for bacterial

67

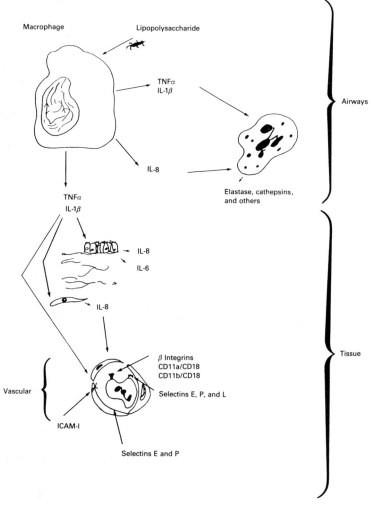

Figure 5.2   A diagram of the cytokine network that controls the migration of neutrophils into the airways. The pulmonary macrophage responds to bacterial products such as lipopolysaccharide by releasing a series of signals in the form of cytokines. IL-8 will increase the numbers of neutrophils in the airways, while TNFα and IL-1β may be important in the activation of primed cells. The same cytokines may act on the epithelial cells that line the airways to induce other cytokines, and on fibroblasts if there is access because of damaged connective tissue and overlying epithelium. These two cell types further release IL-8 which is chemotactic for neutrophils. Under the influence of such cytokines selectins and integrins are expressed.

clearance and is generally more effective against Gram negative than Gram positive organisms. Rat alveolar macrophages exposed in vivo to formalin killed *Ps aeruginosa* release neutrophil chemotactic factors in a dose dependent manner, whereas *in vivo* instillation of the same bacteria leads to pulmonary nutrophilia 24 hours later. The airways (or luminal) macrophage probably has the key role at least in the early stages of infection of coordinating the inflammatory response, although later it is likely that the interstitial macrophage maintains the mucosal inflammatory response and leads to cell mediated tissue injury through neutrophils, monocytes, and T-lymphocytes.

Intravascular pulmonary macrophages provide a link between the lung and the systemic response to infection. This is probably by the release of cytokines, chemotactic factors, and the facilitation of endothelial aspects of cellular transit from the vascular compartment. The intravascular pulmonary macrophage, in particular, is an efficient particle-removing cell[43] and may be an important regulator of circulating immune complexes arising from the lung in cystic fibrosis. The presence of circulating cytokines such as TNFα and interleukins may augment and maintain the inflammatory response[44] and may also mediate the development of the cachexia associated with chronic cystic fibrosis.

Polymorphonuclear neutrophil

Neutrophils are the predominant cells of the airways and lung parenchyma in patients with chronic *Ps aeruginosa* infection, and form a substantial systemic circulatory component in response to lung infection. Cells such as the neutrophil and monocyte are largely recruited from the circulation by chemotactic stimuli. This is shown by increased neutrophil transit into the lung and also the presence of neutrophil granule products in the circulation and airways.[44–47] Granule products such as lactoferrin and elastase probably derive from the intravascular activation of neutrophils as they marginate and migrate into the lung. This occurs in other types of lung injury such as adult respiratory distress syndrome, and may be used to monitor the inflammatory response.[44 46–48] Neutrophils are well equipped both to destroy bacteria and to cause extensive tissue injury. They produce de novo superoxide anion through the NADPH-oxidase system in the plasma membrane of the cell. Superoxide in the presence of halides and myeloperoxidase gives rise to a range of highly active metabolites which are extremely toxic to surrounding cells and cause damage to cell membranes. The neutrophil also contains many enzymatic and cationic products which are also capable of causing extensive injury. The neutrophil is remarkably potent in terms of enzymes that break down the major connective tissue protein found in lungs.[49]

Lymphocytes

Both T and B lymphocytes are likely to play a part in the lung injury associated with cystic fibrosis. Cell mediated tissue injury by T-lymphocytes may occur in the mucosa of the airways. In animal models of psuedomonal infections there is a close association between activated interstitial macrophages and T-lymphocytes.[50] Large amounts of immunoglobulin are produced and directed against antigens derived from the infecting bacteria. Precipitating antibodies to *Staph aureus*, *H influenzae* and *Ps aeruginosa* occur, but their role is largely unclear, particularly for *H influenzae* and *S aureus*. In *Ps aeruginosa* infection there is a massive antibody response to bacterial exoproducts, but later antibodies to cell wall lipopolysaccharide predominate with the formation of immune complexes both within the lung and within the circulation. Early on such antibodies may be protective, particularly if they are opsonically active,[51] whereas in the later phases of the disorder high concentrations of immune complexes form and spill over into the circulation from the lung and indicate the terminal phase of pulmonary inflammation.[52] Immune complexes might maintain the inflammatory response by direct stimulation of various inflammatory cells although immunoglobulins cannot penetrate the alginate coating of *Ps aeruginosa* and are unlikely to be an effective opsonising agent after alginate production has begun. Opsonisation is reduced further because of the production of IgG class II immunoglobulin which has a low opsonic potency.[53] Opsonic capacity is reduced further by cleavage of the crystallisable (Fc) fragment of immunoglobulins by both bacterial elastase and neutrophil elastase, but this may have regulatory advantages as Fc "free" immune complexes do not stimulate the neutrophil oxidative burst.[54] A vicious cycle therefore develops, that works against the interests of the host. This is initiated and maintained by the presence of bacteria and the host response itself becomes a self-perpetuating positively re-enforcing system leading to continuous lung injury.

Cytokine function in cystic fibrosis

A range of cytokines, including IL-1α, IL-1β, IL-6, IL-8, and TNFα may be associated with inflammatory activity in the lung in cystic fibrosis. IL-1β and TNFα act as proximal, or primary, mediators that lead to the development of secondary production of other cytokines and form a network to regulate the inflammatory response. An important network of cytokines may be acting in the mechanisms underlying the regulation of neutrophil migration from the circulation to the lungs.

Control of neutrophil infiltration of the lung in cystic fibrosis

The neutrophil is the main effector cell of injury and its recruitment from the vascular space to the interstitium and airways is paramount to the injury process. A full understanding of these events might indicate useful therapeutic interventions. Recruitment from the circulation includes activation of endothelial cells and the expression of neutrophil adhesion molecules, activation of neutrophils and the expression of endothelium adhesion molecules, neutrophil-endothelial cell adhesion and neutrophil diapedesis and migration within the extravascular space.

Two interacting groups of adhesion molecules are expressed on the cell membrane of the neutrophil; the β-integrins and the selectins. The β-integrin adhesion molecules are a group of heterodimeric glycoproteins expressed only in the plasma membrane of leucocytes. Each molecule comprises two chains, an α-chain with a variable amino acid sequence and a β-chain with a constant sequence. These molecules form functional clusters with the following designations: CD11a/CD18, CD11b/CD18, and CD11c/CD18. Of these, CD11b/CD18 is the major integrin associated with neutrophils and is expressed in a sequestered form in the membrane of secondary and tertiary granules.[55][56] CD11a/CD18 is expressed on all leucocytes, but may be less important for neutrophil adhesion than the CD11b/CD18 β-integrins. Activation of the neutrophil by IL-1β, TNFα, and IL-8, or any combination thereof, leads to a rapid translocation of the CD11b/CD18 molecule to the cell surface.[55][56] The major natural ligands/receptors for this complex are the split product of complement iC3b and the intracellular adhesion molecule 1 (ICAM-1) which is constituently expressed on endothelial cells. The fundamental role of these adhesion molecules has been shown

71

by the use of monoclonal antibodies to either the CD11b or CD18 component which reduce neutrophil dependent vascular permeability in lung injury in animal models.[57-59]

The other group of adhesion molecules expressed on the cell membrane of the neutrophil is the family known as selectins. These are also known as LEC-CAMs (lectin, epidermal growth factor complement, cellular adhesion molecules).[60] L, E, and P-selectins seem to be important in neutrophil adhesion. L-selectin is constitutively expressed on the surface of leucocytes, whilst E-selectin expression is induced by endotoxin, TNFα or IL-1β. P-selectin is expressed on the surface of neutrophils after its release from either platelets or the Weibel-Palade bodies of endothelial cells.[61]

The roles of these two groups of adhesion molecules seem to be slightly different. Selectin molecules are important for interaction with activated endothelial cells as a primary event leading to margination or rolling under high sheer force conditions in the capillary circulation. β-integrins seem to have no role in this early phase of margination but are essential to ensure stable intra-vascular adhesion for trans-endothelial migration.[62]

Endothelial cells constitutively express ICAM-1 which is the major counter receptor for the CD11b/CD18, and CD11a/CD18 β-integrins. Expression of ICAM-1 is also increased by lipopoly-saccharide, TNFα, and IL-1β.[55 56] This molecule is also expressed on the surface of mononuclear phagocytes, fibroblasts, and epithelial cells and may have an important role in the movement of neutrophils through tissue, such as the interstitium of the lung. Neutralising antibodies to the ICAM-1 molecule are as effective as

---

Adhesion molecules

- **β-integrins:** heterodimeric glycoproteins comprising an α chain with a variable amino acid sequence and a β chain with a constant sequence
- **Selectins:** L-selectin expressed on the surface of leucocytes
E-selectin expression induced by endotoxin, TNFα, or IL-1β
P-selectin released from platelets or endothelial cells and expressed on surface of neutrophils

anti-β-integrin monoclonal antibodies in attenuating neutrophil dependent lung injury.

E-selectin is also expressed by endothelial cells in response to lipopolysaccharide, TNFα or IL-1β.[60] The expression of selectins seems to be a rapid and early event compared with the expression of ICAM-1 by endothelial cells. P-selectin is rapidly mobilised to the surface of endothelial cells after it has been exposed to a variety of inflammatory mediators. Expression of both selectins promotes neutrophil adhesion which is dependent upon recognition of the Lewis-X-oligosaccharide associated with the L-selectin molecule.[63] This further emphasises the importance of selectins in the early margination process of neutrophils.

Current understanding of neutrophil and endothelial cell interaction through such adhesion molecules has led to the development of a hypothesis that neutrophil migration is largely under the control of a network of cytokines which therefore primarily regulates the inflammatory process in the lung in cystic fibrosis. The signal for neutrophil migration into the lung progresses from the ingestion of bacteria by pulmonary macrophages, probably in the airways, which synthesise and secrete a range of cytokines including TNFα, IL-1β, IL-6, and IL-8. Other cells, such as epithelial cells and pulmonary fibroblasts, may respond to the stimulation by TNFα and IL-1β to produce more IL-8 and so generate a chemotactic gradient that attracts neutrophils across the extravascular space (Figure 5.2). IL-8 also induces the expression of CD11b/CD18 molecules on the plasma membrane of neutrophils, so IL-8, TNFα, and IL-1β acting together increase the expression of adhesion molecules on both neutrophils and endothelial cells. These effects increase neutrophil adhesion, activation, margination, diapedesis, and extravascular migration.

This hypothesis is based on the concept that TNFα and IL-1β are proximal, or early response, cytokines that regulate the development of distal mediators to form a cytokine network, and is supported by studies of neutrophil migration into the lung from the circulation using intravascular stimulation such as lipopolysaccharide and alveolitis induced by lipopolysaccharide or IL-1β given intratracheally.

TNFα and IL-1β look trophic with many overlapping and some synergistic functions with regard to cellular activity. These effects in the lung in cystic fibrosis are likely to be important regulators of the initiation, maintenance, and severity of tissue injury, as well as localising infection to the lung and initiating the healing process.[64]

73

reatment and prevention

Lung injury occurs from the earliest weeks of life and considerably reduces survival in cystic fibrosis. Currently the main factor changing survival rates is the reduction of mortality in the first year of life. Thereafter survival curves of patients tend to run in parallel with those of the past, but offset by that initial improvement.[1] A positive approach to the protection of the lung from early in life seems to be the only way to change the slope of the survival curve. Greater knowledge of the control of the inflammatory response in the lung in cystic fibrosis would be of considerable advantage as survival with chronic bronchial sepsis is an important burden on resources and greatly reduces the quality of life for survivors. A more subtle approach to controlling specific inflammatory mechanisms at an early stage may halt injury, or at least reduce the rate of progress, leading to better survival and a higher quality of life. In cystic fibrosis treatment with corticosteroids may preserve lung function, though the mechanisms are unknown,[65] and the risk of side effects considerable. Various other potential treatments are being studied. Non-steroidal anti-inflammatory agents, which act by inhibiting cyclooxygenase, reduce lung injury in experimental *Ps aeruginosa* pneumonia in animals,[66] and a four year study of high dose ibuprofen in children and adults with mild lung disease ($FEV_1 > 60\%$ predicted) showed slowing of the decline in lung function and better maintenance of body weight on treatment compared with placebo.[67] The future may yield specific anti-elastase compounds, antioxidants, antagonists for receptors for specific cytokines, monoclonal antibodies to specific cytokines, and agents like pentoxifylline, which have a wide range of anti-inflammatory effects and protect against lethal bacterial infection in animals.[68] Even with knowledge of the cystic fibrosis gene, and the structure of the cystic fibrosis transmembrane regulator protein, many patients are likely to be at risk of shortened life span because of chronic pulmonary infections for several decades to come.

References

1 Elborn JS, Shale DJ, Britton JR. Cystic fibrosis: current survival and population estimates to the year 2000. *Thorax* 1991; **46**: 881–5.
2 Oppenheimer EH, Esterly JR. Pathology of cystic fibrosis. Review of the literature and comparison with 146 autopsied cases. *Prospect Pediatr Pathol* 1978; 2: 241–78.
3 Bedrossian CWM, Greenberg SD, Singer DB, Hansen JJ, Rosenberg HS. The

74

lung in cystic fibrosis. A quantitative study of pathologic findings amongst different age groups. *Hum Pathol* 1976; 7: 195–204.

4 Cole PJ. Inflammation: a two-edged sword – the model of bronchiectasis. *Eur J Respir Dis* 1986; 69: (suppl 147): 6–15.

5 Sykes DA, Wilson R, Greenstone M, Currie DC, Steinfort C, Cole PJ. Deleterious effects of purulent sputum sol on human ciliary function in vitro: at least two factors identified. *Thorax* 1987; 42: 256–61.

6 Baltimore RS, Christie CDC, Walker-Smith GJ. Immunohistopathologic location of *Pseudomonas aeruginosa* in lungs from patients with cystic fibrosis – implications for the pathogenesis of progressive lung deterioration. *Am Rev Respir Dis* 1989; 140: 1650–61.

7 Pedersen NT, Høiby N, Mordhorst CH, Lind K, Flensborg EW, Bruun B. Respiratory infection in cystic fibrosis patients caused by virus, chlamydia and mycoplasma – possible synergism with *Pseudomonas aeruginosa*. *Acta Paediatrica Scandinavica* 1981; 70: 623–8.

8 Abman SH, Ogle LW, Butler-Simon N, Rumack CM, Accurso FJ. Role of respiratory syncitial virus in early hospitalisation for respiratory distress in young infants with cystic fibrosis. *J Pediatr* 1988; 113: 826–30.

9 Efthimiou J, Hodson ME, Taylor P, Taylor AG, Batten JC. Importance of viruses and *Legionella pneumophila* in respiratory exacerbations of young adults with cystic fibrosis. *Thorax* 1984; 39: 150–4.

10 Conway SP, Simmonds EJ, Littlewood JM. Acute severe deterioration in cystic fibrosis associated with Influenza A virus infection. *Thorax* 1992; 47: 112–4.

11 Wang EEL, Prober CG, Manson B, Corey M, Levison H. Association of respiratory viral infections with pulmonary deterioration in patients with cystic fibrosis. *N Engl J Med* 1984; 331: 1653–8.

12 Johansen HK, Høiby N. Seasonal onset of initial colonisation and chronic infection with *Pseudomonas aeruginosa* in Denmark. *Thorax* 1992; 47: 109–11.

13 Lewin LO, Byard PJ, Davis PB. Effects of *Pseudomonas cepacia* colonization on survival and pulmonary function of cystic fibrosis patients. *J Clin Epidemiol* 1990; 43: 125–31.

14 Elborn JS, Cordon SM, Shale DJ. Inflammatory responses to first isolation of *Pseudomonas aeruginosa* from sputum in cystic fibrosis. *Pediatr Pulmonol* 1993; 15: 287–91.

15 Høiby N. Microbiology of lung infections in cystic fibrosis patients. *Acta Paediatrica Scandinavica* 1982; 301: (suppl) 33–54.

16 Ericsson A, Granstrom M, Mollby R, Strandvik B. Antibodies to staphylococcal teichoic acid and alpha toxin in patients with cystic fibrosis. *Acta Paediatrica Scandinavica* 1986; 75: 139–44.

17 Kulczyki LL, Murphy TM, Bellanti JA. Pseudomonas colonisation in cystic fibrosis. A study in 160 patients. *JAMA* 1978; 240: 30–4.

18 Marks MI. The pathogenesis and treatment of pulmonary infections in patients with cystic fibrosis. *J Pediatr* 1981; 98: 173–9.

19 Szaff M, Høiby N. Antibiotic treatment of *Staphylococcus aureus* infection in cystic fibrosis. *Acta Paediatrica Scandinavica* 1982; 71: 821–6.

20 Høiby N, Kilian M. Haemophilus from the lower respiratory tract of patients with cystic fibrosis. *Scand J Respir Dis* 1976; 57: 103–7.

21 Howard AJ, Dunkin KT, Millar GW. Nasopharyngeal carriage and antibiotic resistance of *Haemophilus influenzae* in healthy children. *Epidemiol Infect* 1988; 100: 193–203.

22 Long SS, Teter MJ, Gilligan PH. Biotype of *Haemophilus influenzae*: correlation with virulence and ampicillin resistance. *J Infect Dis* 1983; 147: 800–6.

23 Shann F, Gratten M, Germer D, Linneman V, Hazlett D, Payne R. Aetiology of pneumonia in children in Goroka Hospital, Papua New Guinea. *Lancet* 1984; ii: 537–41.

24 Wilson R, Cole P. Pathogenic mechanisms during infection of the respiratory

75

tract with special reference to *Haemophilus influenzae*. In: Howard AJ, ed. *Haemophilus influenzae: antimicrobials and the host response*. London: Royal College of Medicine Services, 1988: 7–16 (Publication 138).

25 Jankowskie R, Wayoff M, Lion C, Burdin JC, Foliguiet B. Virulence of *Haemophilus influenzae*. In: Rigelmann R, ed. *Update of Haemophilus influenzae; how virulence, incidence and resistance affect treatment*. London: Royal Society of Medicine Services, 1988: 41–48 (Publication 128).

26 Sheinman ZBD, Devalia JL, Davis RJ, Crook S. Synthesis of histamine by *Haemophilus influenzae*. *BMJ* 1986; **292**: 857–8.

27 Rayner RJ, Hiller EJ, Ispahani P, Baker M. Haemophilus infection in cystic fibrosis. *Arch Dis Child* 1990; **65**: 255–8.

28 Roberts DE, Higgs E, Rutman A, Cole P. Isolation of spheroplastic forms of *Haemophilus influenzae* from sputum in conventionally treated chronic bronchial sepsis using selective medium supplemented with N-acetyle-D-glucosamine: possible reservoir for re-emergence of infection. *BMJ* 1984; **289**: 1409–12.

29 Roberts DE, Cole P. Use of selective media in bacteriological investigation of patients with chronic suppurative respiratory infection. *Lancet* 1980; **i**: 786–7.

30 Høiby N, Koch C. *Pseudomonas aeruginosa* infection in cystic fibrosis and its management. *Thorax* 1990; **45**: 881–4.

31 Kerem E, Corey M, Gold R, Levison H. Pulmonary function and clinical course in patients with cystic fibrosis after pulmonary colonisation with *Pseudomonas aeruginosa*. *J Pediatr* 1990; **116**: 714–9.

32 Theander TG, Kharazmi A, Pedersen BK, Christensen LD, Tvede N, Poulson LK, *et al.* Inhibition of luman lymphocyte proliferation and cleavage of interleukin-2 by *Pseudomonas aeruginosa* proteases. *Infect Immun* 1988; **56**: 1673–7.

33 Nutman J, Berger M, Chase PA *et al.* Studies on the mechanism of T-cell inhibition by the *Pseudomonas aeruginosa* phenzine pigment pyocyanin. *J Immunol* 1987; **138**: 3481–7.

34 Muhlradt PF, Tsai H, Conradt P. Effect of pyocyanine, a blue pigment from *Pseudomonas aeruginosa*, on separate steps of T-cell activation: interleukin-2 (IL-2) production, IL-2 receptor formation, proliferation and induction of cytolytic activity. *Eur J Immunol* 1986; **16**: 434–40.

35 Heath AW. Cytokines and infection. *Curr Opin Immunol* 1990; **2**: 380–4.

36 Horvat RT, Parmely MJ. *Pseudomonas aeruginosa* alkaline protease degrades human gamma interferon and inhibits its bioactivity. *Infect Immun* 1988; **56**: 2925–32.

37 Horvat RT, Clabaugh M, Duval-Jobe C, Parmely MJ. Inactivation of human gamma interferon by *Pseudomonas aeruginosa* proteases; elastase augments the effects of alkaline protease despite the presence of α_1-macroglobulin. *Infect Immun* 1989; **57**: 1668–74.

38 Parmely M, Gale A, Glabaugh M, Horvat RT, Zhou W-W. Proteolytic inactivation of cytokines by *Pseudomonas aeruginosa*. *Infect Immun* 1990; **58**: 3009–14.

39 Novelli F, Giovarelli M, Reber-Liske R, Virgallita G, Garotta G, Forni G. Blockade of physiologically secreted IFN-γ inhibits human T lymphocyte and natural killer cell activation. *J Immunol* 1991; **147**: 1445-52.

40 Kunkel SL, Standiford T, Kasahara K, Strieter RM. Interleukin-8 (IL-8): the major neutrophil chemotactic factor in the lung. *Exp Lung Res* 1991; **17**: 17–23.

41 Sibille Y, Reynolds HY. Macrophages and polymorphonuclear neutrophils in lung defence and injury. *Am Rev Respir Dis* 1990; **41**: 471–501.

42 Ozaki T, Maeda M, Hayashi H, *et al.* Role of alveolar macrophages in the neutrophil dependent defence system against *Pseudomonas aeruginosa* infection in the lower respiratory tract. *Am Rev Respir Dis* 1989; **140**: 1595–1601.

43 Dehring DJ, Mismar BL. Intravascular macrophages in pulmonary capillaries of

humans. *Am Rev Respir Dis* 1989; **139**: 1027–9.

44 Suter S, Schaad UB, Roux-Lombard P, Girardin E, Grau G, Dayer JM. Relation between tumour necrosis factor-α and granulocyte elastase-α_1 proteinase inhibitor complexes in the plasma of patients with cystic fibrosis. *Am Rev Respir Dis* 1989; **140**: 1640–4.

45 Currie DC, Saverymurru SH, Petters AM *et al.* Indium-III-labelled granulocyte accumulation in respiratory tract of patients with bronchiectasis. *Lancet* 1987; **ii**: 1335–8.

46 Rayner RJ, Wiseman MS, Cordon SM, Norman D, Hiller EJ, Shale DJ. Inflammatory markers in cystic fibrosis. *Respir Med* 1991; **85**: 139–45.

47 Norman D, Elborn JS, Cordon SM, Wiseman MS, Rayner RJ, Hiller EJ *et al.* Plasma tumour necrosis factor-alpha in cystic fibrosis. *Thorax* 1991; **46**: 91–5.

48 Rocker GM, Wiseman MS, Pearson D, Shale DJ. Diagnostic criteria for adult respiratory distress syndrome: time; time for reappraisal. *Lancet* 1989; **ii**: 120–3.

49 Borregaard N. Bactericidal mechanisms of the human neutrophil. *Scand J Haematol* 1984; **32**: 225–30.

50 Lappa e Silva JR, Guerreiro D, Noble B, Poulter LW, Cole PJ. Immunopathology of experimental bronchiectasis. *Am J Respir Cell Mol Biol* 1989; **1**: 297–304.

51 Pier GB, Saunders JM, Ames P *et al.* Opsonophagic killing antibody to *Pseudomonas aeruginosa* mucoid exo-polysaccharide in older non-colonised patients with cystic fibrosis. *N Engl J Med* 1987; **317**: 793–8.

52 Dasgupta MK, Lam JS, Döring G, *et al.* Prognostic implications of circulating immune complexes and *Pseudomonas aeruginosa* specific antibodies in cystic fibrosis. *J Clin Lab Immunol* 1987; **23**: 25–30.

53 Pressler T, Mausa B, Jensen T, Pedersen SS, Høiby N. Increased IgG, and IgG concentration is associated with advanced *Pseudomonas aeruginosa* infection and poor pulmonary function in cystic fibrosis. *Acta Paediatrica Scandinavica* 1988; **77**: 576–82.

54 Döring G, Goldstein W, Botzenhart K, Kharazmi A. Elastase from polymorphonuclear leucocytes: a regulatory enzyme in immune complex disease. *Clin Exp Immunol* 1986; **64**: 597–605.

55 Arnaout MA. Structure and function of the leukocyte adhesion molecules CD11/SC18. *Blood* 1990; **75**: 1037–50.

56 Springer TA. Adhesion receptors of the immune system. *Nature* 1990; **346**: 425–34.

57 Vedder NB, Winn RK, Rice CL, Chi EY, Arfars KE, Harlan JM. A monoclonal antibody to the adherence-promoting leukocyte glycoprotein CD18, reduces organ injury and improves survival from hemorrhagic shock and resuscitation in rabbits. *J Clin Invest* 1988; **81**: 939–44.

58 Mulligan MS, Varani J, Warren JS, Till GO, Smith CW, Anderson DC, *et al.* Roles of β_2 integrins of rate neutrophils in complement-and oxygen radical-mediated acute inflammatory injury. *J Immunol* 1992; **148**: 1447–57.

59 Mulligan MS, Warren JS, Smith CW, Anderson DC, Yeh CG, Rudolph AR, *et al.* Lung injury after deposition of IgA immune complexes; requirements for CD18 and L-arginine. *J Immunol* 1992; **148**: 3086–92.

60 Lasky LA. Lectin cell adhesion molecules (LEC-CAMs); a new family of cell adhesion proteins involved with inflammation. *J Cell Biochem* 1991; **45**: 139–46.

61 McEver RP, Beckstead JH, Moore KL, Marshall-Carlson L, Bainton DF. HMP-140, a platelet alpha-granule membrane protein, is also synthesized by vascular endothelial cells and is localized in Weibel-Palade bodies. *J Clin Invest* 1989; **84**: 92–7.

62 Butcher EC. Leukocyte-endothelial cell recognition; three (or more) steps to specificity and diversity. *Cell* 1991; **67**: 1033–6.

63 Picker LJ, Warnock RA, Burns A, Doerschuk CM, Berg EL, Butcher EC. The neutrophil selectin LECAM-1 presents carbohydrate ligands to the vascular selectins ELAM-1 and GMP-140. *Cell* 1991; **66**: 921–33.
64 Le J, Vilceck J. TNF and IL-1: cytokines with multiple overlapping biological activities. *Lab Invest* 1987; **56**: 234–82.
65 Auerbach HS, Williams M, Kirkpatrick JA, Cotten HR. Alternate-day prednisolone reduces morbidity and improves pulmonary function in cystic fibrosis. *Lancet* 1985; **ii**: 686–8.
66 Konstan MW, Vargo KM, Davis PB. Ibuprofen attenuates the inflammatory response to *Pseudomonas aeruginosa* in a rat model of chronic pulmonary infection. *Am Rev Respir Dis* 1990; **141**: 186–92.
67 Konstan MW, Bigard PJ, Hoppel CL, David PB. Effect of high-dose ibuprofen in patients with cystic fibrosis. *N Engl J Med* 1995; **332**: 845–54.
68 Ishizaka A, Wu Z, Stephens FE, *et al.* Attenuation of acute lung injury in septic guinea pigs by pentoxifylline. *Am Rev Respir Dis* 1988; **318**: 376–82.

6 Infection

NIELS HØIBY, CHRISTIAN KOCH

Patients with cystic fibrosis have no detectable immune deficiency and, except for the respiratory tract, they are no more susceptible to infection than other children of the same age; indeed, bacteraemia is rarely recorded in patients with cystic fibrosis.[1] The altered secretions in the respiratory tract that lead to thick mucus are thought to be the primary reason for the recurrent and chronic respiratory tract infections seen in cystic fibrosis. It can therefore be regarded as a disorder that is associated with a serious defect in the primary, non-specific defence mechanism of the respiratory tract — the mucociliary escalator defence.

Acute exacerbations of chronic respiratory disease in patients with cystic fibrosis have been found to be caused by bacteria alone (63%), bacteria plus viruses (13%), and viruses alone (6%), whereas no aetiological factor was found in only 18% of exacerbations.[2] Prevention of such infections is the main potential outcome of correcting the basic defect in the respiratory tract by gene therapy.

Respiratory viral infections

Respiratory viruses including influenza viruses A and B, parainfluenza viruses 1 and 3, rhinovirus, adenovirus, and particularly respiratory syncytial virus, are responsible for some of the acute exacerbations of pulmonary disease in cystic fibrosis.[2 3-9] As a consequence, pulmonary function may decrease by up to 30% for about a month after a viral infection,[8] and there is a susceptibility to secondary colonisation and infection with bacteria, notably *Pseudomonas aeruginosa*, after such infections.[2 10] Despite the detrimental effect of viral infections, vaccination against influenza

A is the only generally used prophylactic measure and treatment with amantadine or ribavarin is rarely given.[4 11]

Bacterial infections

Some of the major bacterial pathogens in the lungs — for example, *Streptococcus pneumoniae*, *Haemophilus influenzae*, and *Staphylococcus aureus* — are part of the normal flora of the mouth, though in small numbers. Other bacteria such as enterobacteriaceae and *Pseudomonas* species are seldom, if ever, found in the normal flora, though *Escherichia coli* and *Candida albicans* may colonise the mouth after treatment with broad spectrum antibacterial agents which eradicate the sensitive normal flora. The insidious nature of some of the lower respiratory tract infections in cystic fibrosis makes frequent cultures (one or two a month) of sputum or tracheal secretions necessary.

Chronic pulmonary infection with *Ps aeruginosa* is defined as persistence of bacteria in respiratory tract secretions for six months or more, or development of an appreciable antibody response, or both.[12] Antibody responses to *Ps aeruginosa* and other bacteria (*Staph aureus*, *H influenzae*, *Burkholderia cepacia*, and others if they are isolated repeatedly from sputum) are measured in some cystic fibrosis centres routinely at least once a year to rule out undetected chronic infection, or more often if the patient's condition deteriorates.[12] IgG and IgE antibodies to *Aspergillus fumigatus* are also measured in patients with suspected allergic bronchopulmonary aspergillosis.[13–16]

Bacteria remain the most important micro-organisms responsible for the progression of the lung disease,[17–19] with *Ps aeruginosa* being associated with 51% of acute exacerbations, *Staph aureus* with 19%, *H influenzae* with 14%, *Strep pneumoniae* with 5%, and enterobacteriaceae with 10%.[2] In young children the bacteria most commonly involved are *Staph aureus* and *H influenzae*, but pneumococci and sometimes enterobacteriaceae are also isolated (Table 6.1).[12 20] In older children and adults these bacteria may still have a role, but the main pathogen is *Ps aeruginosa* and in some centres *B cepacia* and other pathogens as well.[12 20] The tendency for *Staph aureus*, *H influenzae*, and *Strep pneumoniae* to cause mainly recurrent infections, and for *Ps aeruginosa*, *B cepacia*, and mycobacteria to cause mainly chronic infections, may reflect differences in the efficacy of chemotherapy.[2] Anaerobic infections are not a serious problem in cystic fibrosis.

Table 6.1   Point prevalence rate (%) of the major bacterial pathogens in 192 patients with cystic fibrosis treated in the Danish Centre, 1984.

Bacterial species	Prevalence (%) in different age groups (years)			
	0–9	10–19	≥20	Total
Staph aureus	55	35	30	42
H influenzae	30	9	8	17
Strep pneumoniae	21	1	3	10
E coli	10	1	8	6
Ps aeruginosa	25	81	81	57

Modified from Pedersen et al.[20]

Staphylococcus aureus

Since the original description of cystic fibrosis *Staph aureus* has been considered to be an important pathogen, though no immune deficiency to these bacteria have been described (Table 6.1).[12 21] Its particularly close association with cystic fibrosis has been ascribed to the high electrolyte content, the changed composition of lipids in sputum in cystic fibrosis, the presence of a polysaccharide capsule, or the effect of protein A as an IgG scavenger.[12 22 23] No specific phage type is characteristic of infection with *Staph aureus* in cystic fibrosis.[12, 23] It is still the most common pathogen isolated in children with cystic fibrosis, but because of the efficacy of current antibiotics it is no longer a problem. In some centres, however, it remains a cause of considerable numbers of chronic infections but these do not lead to increased mortality as they did in the preantibiotic era.[12] Infection with *Staph aureus* may cause some of the early damage to the respiratory tract in infants and increase the chance of infection with *Ps aeruginosa*.[12 24] Based on this hypothesis, some cystic fibrosis centres prescribe prophylactic antibiotics against *Staph aureus* throughout childhood. Others, such as the Danish centre, attempt to eradicate it whenever it is present in the lower respiratory tract (see Boxes).[25–9] The result of such an aggressive approach is that chronic *Staph aureus* infection seldom occurs in such centres.[12]

There are few controlled clinical studies that compared on demand antistaphylococcal treatment and prophylaxis regimens, though oral antistaphylococcal prophylaxis was shown to be beneficial when compared with inhalation.[29–30] The principles and drugs used in the Danish cystic fibrosis centre are shown in the boxes. Oral treatment is preferred and saves the patients having to be admitted to hospital for treatment. Microbiological efficacy in

---

Specific principles of chemotherapy of lung infections in patients with cystic fibrosis[17]

- *Staph aureus, H influenzae,* and *Ps aeruginosa** — Should be eradicated when present in the lower respiratory tract whether there are clinical symptoms or not
- *Ps aeruginosa*** — two precipitating antibodies against *Ps aeruginosa* means chronic infection and chemotherapy is given regularly at least four times a year
- *B cepacia* — Continuous suppressive treatment with antibiotics given orally; acute exacerbations are treated with antibiotics, given intravenously or by aerosol
- Other pathogens — Seldom pathogenic in cystic fibrosis; chemotherapy is given when indicated by clinical or serological findings. Allergic bronchopulmonary aspergillosis is treated with steroid hormones even if the patient is colonised with other pathogens

* Intermittently colonised; ** chronically colonised.

---

terms of eradication does not decrease and remains at about 75% with bacterial resistance occurring only rarely.[31] If treatment fails, four weeks' treatment with one of the combinations of antibiotics given orally (Box) and sometimes inhaled methicillin is used. Other less aggressive regimens and the basis of rational selection and doses of antistaphylococcal antibiotics have been described.[18 21 25 32-4]

Haemophilus influenzae

Most strains of *H influenzae* that are isolated from the respiratory tract in patients with cystic fibrosis are non-capsulated, and no deficiency in host defence against these bacteria has been described.[12 21 35-6] These bacteria are probably responsible for some acute exacerbations of respiratory symptoms and in a few patients chronic *H influenzae* infection develops.[24] Because of the frequent use of ampicillin and other β-lactam antibiotics, β-lactamase-producing strains are often isolated from sputum. In the Danish cystic fibrosis centre 10%–20% of the strains are β-lactamase producers and have emerged during treatment with ampicillin or amoxycillin.[37] Combinations of ampicillin or amoxycillin with β-lactamase inhibitors, or the use of other drugs such as the fluoroquinolones, are effective in such cases.[38] As with *Staph aureus* there are few reports of controlled studies that compare different

Antibiotics used to treat lung infections in patients with cystic fibrosis.[17 38]

- *Staph aureus* — Dicloxacillin 25 mg/kg/24 h orally + fusidic acid 50 mg/kg/24 h; drugs which can replace one of the above mentioned are rifampicin 15 mg/kg/24 h, and clindamycin 20–40 mg/kg/24 h
- *H influenzae* — Pivampicillin 35 mg/kg/24 h orally or amoxycillin 25–50 mg/kg/24 h; other drugs: amoxacillin + clavulanate (50 mg + 12.5 mg/kg/24 h) *or* rifampicin (15 mg/kg/24 h) combined with erythromycin 30–50 mg/kg/24 h
- *B cepacia* — Doxycycline 100 mg/24 h orally as continuous suppressive treatment. Acute exacerbations are treated with: Co-trimoxazole 100 + 20 mg/kg/24 h orally or intravenously; *or* meropenem 120 mg/kg/24 h *or* chloramphenicol 50–100 mg/kg/24 h orally (maximum 3 g/24 h for 14 days) *or* tobramycin 10–20 mg/kg/24 h intravenously + ceftazidime 150–250 mg/kg/24 h *and/or* ceftazidime 2–4 g/24 h by aerosol; *and/or* rifampicin 15 mg/kg/24 h orally;
- *Ps aeruginosa** — Ciprofloxacin 20–30 mg/kg/24 h orally + colistin 2–3 million units/24 h by aerosol
- *Ps aeruginosa*** — Tobramycin 10–20(–30) mg/kg/24 h intravenously + Piperacillin 300 mg/kg/24 h; *or* + cefsulodin 100–150 mg/kg/24 h; *or* + ceftazidime 150–250 mg/kg/24 h; *or* + aztreonam 150–250 mg/kg/24 h; *or* + Imipenem 50–75 mg/kg/24 h; *or* meropenem 120 mg/kg/24 h; *and* + colistin 2–4 million units/24 h by aerosol *and/or* + ciprofloxacin 20–40 mg/kg/24 h
- Probenecid is given orally to all patients receiving β-lactam antibiotics eliminated by tubular excretion
- Dose of other antibiotics for aerosol treatment: tobramycin: 200 mg/24 h; ceftazidime: 2–4 g/24 h

* Intermittently colonised; ** Chronically colonised.

regimens of treatment of *H influenzae*, and the policy of the Danish cystic fibrosis centre is given in the boxes. Treatment is with antibiotics given orally and the efficacy of bacterial eradication with repeated courses of treatment remains at about 75%.[39] When treatment fails, repeated treatment (sometimes for four weeks) with one of the combinations given in the box, with ciprofloxacin or ofloxacin is used. With this regimen less than 10% of Danish patients are chronically infected (continuously for six months or more) and antibody responses are low.[39] Other less aggressive regimens and the basis for rational selection and doses of antihaemophilus antibiotics for patients with cystic fibrosis have been described.[18 21 32-3]

Burkholderia cepacia

This Gram negative, motile rod occurs in the environment, mainly in soil, and is a pathogen for vegetables. It is seldom isolated from human infections and is rarely found as a nosocomial pathogen in patients who do not have cystic fibrosis. The species emerged as a pathogen in cystic fibrosis about 20 years ago, and has become endemic in some large centres; recently it has occurred as an epidemic species in other centres.[40-53]

The prevalence of *B cepacia* varies widely,[54 55] but overall prevalence is low at 3.2% in the United States in 1990 compared with the 60.7% prevalence of *Ps aeruginosa*.[56] Its prevalence in the first year of life was 0.5%, increasing to 3.4%–5.75% in adult patients.[56] One reason for the difference in prevalence among centres seems to be cross-infection, which has been described in cystic fibrosis centres in Cleveland and elsewhere, but not in other centres.[55 57-60] Isolation of patients prevented further spread of the bacterium in Cleveland.[57]

Recently *B cepacia* has spread among patients in some European cystic fibrosis centres,[50 55 60] and spread outside centres among patients during social contact has been reported.[51] There are three distinct clinical patterns:

- Chronic asymptomatic carriage either alone or in combination with *Ps aeruginosa*
- Progressive deterioration over several months with recurrent episodes of fever, progressive weight loss, and repeated admissions to hospital
- Rapid, usually fatal, deterioration in patients who had previously had only mild disease.[40 42 45 50]

B cepacia is more resistant to antibiotics than *Ps aeruginosa* and resistance develops easily,[28 61-65] making eradication of the infection virtually impossible by antibiotics (see Boxes). Chronic suppression with doxycycline or cotrimoxazole may improve clinical symptoms, but as no controlled study has been undertaken it is difficult to ascribe the improvement to causality or covariation.[54] In the Danish cystic fibrosis centre patients infected with *B cepacia* are segregated from other patients with cystic fibrosis both within the centre and outside; the incidence and prevalence of *B cepacia* has always been low and no cross-infection has been detected.[54]

Pseudomonas aeruginosa

This Gram negative, motile rod is found particularly in fresh water and soil that has been contaminated by animals or humans.

Poorly chlorinated swimming pools or Jacuzzis may become contaminated. *Ps aeruginosa* is rarely found in the stools of normal people, and then in only small numbers. The most prevalent and severe chronic lung infection in cystic fibrosis is caused by *Ps aeruginosa*,[12 18 19] which has become endemic in patients with cystic fibrosis all over the world. In addition to the lungs, the sinuses[66] and subsequently the gastrointestinal tract[67-8] are often colonised

---

The pathogenesis of chronic *Ps aeruginosa* infection in cystic fibrosis: immune complex mediated tissue damage

Stage of infection	Mechanisms and pathogenesis	Clinical signs
Acquisition[10 78]	Cross-infection Concomitant virus infection	None Acute exacerbation
Attachment[84 86]	Pili, haemagglutinin, exotoxin S, alginate	None
Initial persistent colonisation[173]	Bacterial toxins including: elastase, alkaline protease, exotoxins A and S, phospholipase, lipase	None or minimal
Chronic infection[113]	Persistence: microcolonies embedded in alginate. PMN-pseudomonas mismatch Tissue damage: immune complexes, PMN elastase, cytokines	Chronic suppurative lung inflammation, progressive loss of lung function
Modifying mechanisms[120 174-6]	PMN elastase cleaves immune complexes Increase in antibodies to *Ps aeruginosa*, particularly of IgG_2 and IgG_3 subclasses D508 homozygotes compared with other mutations	Individual clinical course of the infection

PMN = Polymorphonuclear neutrophil leucocyte

by these bacteria. A seasonal pattern of initial colonisation and the onset of chronic infection was observed during a 25 year period with two thirds occurring between October and March and coinciding with the seasonal occurrence of respiratory viral infections.[10] Infection with respiratory syncytial virus may predispose to chronic *Ps aeruginosa* infection.[69]

Acquisition

Patients infected with *Ps aeruginosa* are not infectious to members of their families who do not have cystic fibrosis, but siblings with the disease often carry the same strain indicating cross-infection of colonisation from the same environmental source.[70] Environmental sources have been identified in cystic fibrosis centres, on dental equipment, and in a hydrotherapy pool,[71-76] but studies from holiday camps for patients with cystic fibrosis indicate that the risk of cross-infection is low.[77 78] Large centres have a higher prevalence of *Ps aeruginosa* infection than smaller centres.[78] The mean prevalence of *Ps aeruginosa* infections among patients with cystic fibrosis in the United States was 60.7%; it was 20.8% among the 0–1 year old patients rising to 80.1% among those 30–35 years old.[56]

Cross-infection has occurred in the Danish cystic fibrosis centre[71 78] and some other centres have also indicated the possibility of cross-infection, whereas others could not identify evidence of nosocomial infection.[71 72 74 79-81] By improving the general hygiene of the centre and by segregating infected and uninfected patients – both in different wards and in different outpatient clinics on different days – cross-infection was prevented in the Danish centre.[71 78] The yearly incidence of new chronic infections with *Ps aeruginosa* was reduced to the "natural background" level which is assumed to be 1%–2% a year;[78] the efficacy of segregation has also been reported from another centre.[80] The mean age at acquisition of chronic infection with *Ps aeruginosa* at the Danish centre has risen from 6 to 15 years during the past decade.[82]

Adhesion

Whether colonisation of the upper respiratory tract precedes bronchial infection with *Ps aeruginosa* is unknown; it shows chemotaxis towards mucin-rich mucosal surfaces[83] and in animal studies has been shown to adhere to epithelial cells in the buccal mucosa, the nasal turbinates, and tracheobronchial mucosa as well as to mucus.[84 85] Four types of adhesion factors have been identified on *Ps aeruginosa* — pili, alginate, and possibly haemagglutinin and exotoxin S — which bind to corresponding receptors on the host cells — glycolipids, glycosphingolipids, and glycoproteins that contain lactosyl and sialosyl residues.[84-7] Injury to epithelial cells by trypsin or human leucocyte elastase exposed new receptors for pili and increased bacterial adhesion[84 87] and may increase the risk of bacterial colonisation.

Initial persistent colonisation

In more than 80% of patients a median period of 12 months of intermittent colonisation precedes persistent colonisation.[10] Factors that probably enhance the transition to persistent colonisation (in addition to viral infection) are exotoxins produced by *Ps aeruginosa*, but this point of view is supported by circumstantial evidence alone. *Ps aeruginosa* produces many toxins and virulence factors,[82] some of which may act during establishment of the initial persistent colonisation of the respiratory tract; these include elastase and alkaline protease, which can inhibit non-specific (phagocytes) and immunologically specific (T cells and natural killer cells) defence mechanisms.[88 89] Lipopolysaccharide and alginate may also be important because antibodies to these products can be detected before infection becomes chronic.[82 90] Later the importance of the toxins is doubtful, because specific antibodies are produced and free elastase and alkaline protease can be detected in bronchial secretions only during the first few months of the infection, before neutralising antibodies have developed.[91-3]

Chronic infection

Alginate is the only antigen which correlates with poor prognosis in cystic fibrosis[94-5] and is a characteristic feature of persistent infection when it forms microcolonies in the airways.[18 96-99] The microcolony or biofilm form of growth is a survival strategy of environmental bacteria[100] and the main component of the matrix of the microcolony is alginate (Figure 6.1).[101] Mucoid strains may occur in other patients who are chronically colonised by *Ps aeruginosa*, but such strains are characteristic of cystic fibrosis.[102] *Ps aeruginosa* growing in vitro in alginate biofilms is highly resistant to antibiotics, probably because the organism grows slowly, penetration of the antibiotic is impaired,[102 103] and the organisms are protected against phagocytes and complement.[101 104] Production of β-lactamase is the main mechanism of resistance of *Ps aeruginosa* to

87

β-lactam antibiotics in vivo in cystic fibrosis.[105] In most patients non-mucoid strains initiate the infection and the transition to the mucoid variant occurs with the development of the antibody response to virtually all antigens and exotoxins of *Ps aeruginosa*.[94 106-7] This is of clinical importance as mucoid variants correlate with poor prognosis.[94-5]

Deposition of complement on the surface of mucoid microcolonies may be deficient in patients with cystic fibrosis[108] which favours the survival of such colonies though the embedded bacteria are unusual in other aspects. They are often serum sensitive[109] and polyagglutinable,[110] they may lack the lipopolysaccharide side chain,[111] they are not motile, and they express iron-regulated outer membrane proteins indicating that they grow under iron-restricted conditions in the lungs in cystic fibrosis.[112 113] Polyagglutinability is caused by the semi-rough nature of the lipopolysaccharide and the presence of a common A band of lipopolysaccharide, which seems to be related to bacteriophages that are present in the sputum of patients with cystic fibrosis.[110 114-116] The semi-rough nature of the lipopolysaccharide in strains of *Ps aeruginosa* from patients with cystic fibrosis accords with in vitro results from *Ps aeruginosa* grown

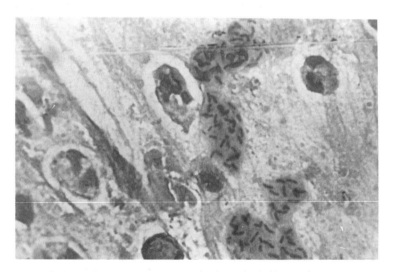

Figure 6.1   Gram-stained smear of sputum from a patient with cystic fibrosis. There is a mucoid microcolony of *Ps aeruginosa* and some polymorphonuclear leucocytes.

in biofilm and with changes in their hydrophobicity.[117]

Lipolysaccharide is the main antigen component of immune complexes in the sputum of patients with chronic *Ps aeruginosa* infection.[118] This unique adaptability to the environment in the lung in cystic fibrosis is reflected in the high incidence of development of antibiotic resistance during chemotherapy. The most striking aspect of the host's response to the infection is the pronounced antibody response which continues to increase for several years and which correlates with poor prognosis. These antibodies are eventually directed against most if not all antigens of *Ps aeruginosa* and they belong to all classes and subclasses of immunoglobulins. Genetically determined individual differences between the IgG subclass antibody response (high IgG2 and IgG3 responses) are, however, correlated with more severe lung infection.[82 119] The correlation between the antibody response and poor prognosis is the result of chronic inflammation mediated by immune complexes in the lungs of patients with cystic fibrosis.[120–122] The inflammatory reaction is dominated by polymorphonuclear leucocytes, and released leucocyte proteases, myeloperoxidase, and oxygen free radicals are the main mechanisms of damage to the lung tissue (Box) (see chapter 5).[123–125]

Vaccination of uninfected patients with a polyvalent *Ps aeruginosa* vaccine was unsuccessful and was associated with a deterioration in lung function that was more rapid than usual.[126] This was probably because it resulted in tissue damage mediated by immune complexes that was similar to that which occurs during chronic infection. Other vaccines are now being evaluated and it is to be hoped that they will provide beneficial effects without immunological side effects if colonisation with *Ps aeruginosa* is not prevented.[127–131] Immunotherapy is currently being evaluated as adjuvant treatment, based on the work of Moss who suggested that a shift from non-opsonising to opsonising antibodies can be obtained by giving passive antibody treatment.[132] Some effect has been found in short term trials, but the risk is similar to that of trials of vaccines in that some patients may experience aggravation of the immune complex disease.

A trial at the Danish cystic fibrosis centre showed that the onset of chronic *Ps aeruginosa* could be prevented or at least delayed by early treatment of the intermittent colonisation with ciprofloxacin given orally and colistin by inhalation for three weeks.[133] In this way *Ps aeruginosa* is treated according to the same principles that are used for the treatment of *Staph aureus* and *H influenzae*, and this regimen is now used routinely at the centre.

Treatment of chronic *Ps aeruginosa* infection is controversial and not particularly successful from a microbiological point of view.[26 27 134 135] In the Danish centre poor prognosis is associated with chronic *Ps aeruginosa* inflection (continuous colonisation for six months or more), and 51% of acute exacerbations of respiratory symptoms were associated with chronic infection.[12] Acute exacerbations are, however, also caused by other pathogens including viruses,[8 12 134 136–8] so the effect of antibiotic treatment for acute exacerbations of chronic *Ps aeruginosa* infection gives conflicting results. There is no consensus, however, about the importance of *Ps aeruginosa* in the prognosis of patients with cystic fibrosis.[134 135] Unfortunately most published trials of chemotherapy have included too few patients resulting in a large type II (β) error.[136 138] In a carefully controlled study antipseudomonas chemotherapy led to a reduced bacterial load in the lungs and improvement in pulmonary function which correlated with this reduction, and the improvement could not be obtained by physiotherapy alone, though the number of patients studied was again small.[136]

In the Danish cystic fibrosis centre another approach has been developed — "maintenance" chemotherapy or "chronic suppressive" chemotherapy.[139] The principle is to suppress the number and activity of the *Ps aeruginosa* bacteria in patients' lungs. This approach has proved to be superior to "on demand" treatment of acute exacerbations, and more than 90% of patients survive for at least 10 years after the onset of chronic infection. This is in contrast to earlier periods when "on demand" treatment resulted in survival of only half at five years.[139–140]

Chronic suppressive treatment is based on the observation that lung function improves during treatment with antibiotics and this effect is still detectable one to two months after the course of treatment. The aim is to restore lung function by repeated regular two week courses of antibiotics given intravenously every three months. The treatment is intensified in patients whose clinical condition is less stable by adding daily inhalations of colistin, and sometimes ciprofloxacin orally as well (Box). The pharmacokinetics of many antibiotics are changed in cystic fibrosis[33] and so higher doses than normal are used because the effect on lung function is dependent on the serum concentrations, particularly of tobramycin.[141] Probenecid is used in many centres to delay the renal excretion of β-lactam antibiotics.[39 142] Outpatient treatment with inhaled aminoglycosides and β-lactam antibiotics with or without ciprofloxacin orally is a regimen used in some centres to avoid admission to hospital.[143 145]

Despite good results it is an expensive regimen and repeated courses of antibiotics cause side effects. Many patients become allergic to some of the β-lactam antibiotics,[146 148] and strains of *Ps aeruginosa* easily become resistant to some of the antibiotics.[149 152] Surprisingly few side effects were recorded during treatment with tobramycin despite repeated high dose courses over many years, but loss of high tone hearing is becoming a problem for some patients.[153] The psychological impact of the intensive treatment and of patients being treated in different groups does not seem to have been too much according to their experience.

Other pathogens

Many other pathogens may colonise the lower respiratory tracts of patients with cystic fibrosis. *Strep pneumoniae* was associated with 5%, and enterobacteriaceae with 10%, of acute exacerbations of respiratory symptoms in patients at the Danish cystic fibrosis centre,[2] but no specific serotypes were identified. *Strep pneumoniae* never causes chronic infections, whereas mucoid strains of *Klebsiella* species, *E coli*, *Citrobacter* species, and even *Proteus* species do.[14] To distinguish between superficial colonisation and chronic infection at the Danish centre they used the antibody response to the offending pathogen (Box). *Legionella pneumophila* is difficult to identify as a pathogen in cystic fibrosis because serological cross reactions with *Ps aeruginosa* invalidate the interpretation of antibody titres.[5 154] *Pasteurella multocida*, *Alcaligenes faecalis*, and *Stenotrophomonas maltophilia* occasionally colonise,[12, 52] and atypical mycobacteria have been detected, but their clinical importance is uncertain in most cases and the results of treatment with antibiotics are disappointing.[155-160] *Mycoplasma pneumoniae* and *Chlamydia* species have no particular importance in cystic fibrosis.[2] *Aspergillus fumigatus* is commonly isolated from the sputum of patients and 5%–10% of them develop acute bronchopulmonary aspergillosis.[161-170] This condition is treated with corticosteroids as in other patients, and sometimes also with antifungal agents.[162 167 171] The importance of *Candida albicans* and related species is uncertain.[15]

In conclusion, more knowledge about the pathology of recurrent and chronic infections and intensive treatment has allowed us to improve the survival and quality of life for patients with cystic fibrosis.[172] Many patients will probably be treated in adult clinics for chest diseases, and it is to be hoped that the principles that we have described can be adapted and refined to improve their quality of life further.

References

1 Fahy JV, Keoghan MT, Crummy EJ, Fitzgerald MX. Bacteraemia and fungaemia in adults with cystic fibrosis. *J Infect* 1991; **22**: 241–5.

2 Petersen NT, Høiby N, Mordhorst C-H, Lind K, Flensborg EW, Bruun B. Respiratory infections in cystic fibrosis caused by virus, chlamydia and mycoplasma – possible synergism with Pseudomonas aeruginosa. *Acta Paediatrica Scandinavica* 1981; **70**: 623–8.

3 Efthimiou J, Hodson ME, Taylor P, Batten JC. Importance of viruses and Legionella pneumophila in respiratory exacerbations of young adults with cystic fibrosis. *Thorax* 1984; **39**: 150–4.

4 Prober CG. The impact of respiratory viral infections in patients with cystic fibrosis. *Clin Rev Allergy* 1991; **9**: 87–102.

5 Ramsey BW, Gore EJ, Smith AL, Cooney MK, Redding GJ, Foy H. The effect of respiratory viral infections on patients with cystic fibrosis. *Am J Dis Child* 1989; **143**: 662–8.

6 Abman SH, Ogle JW, Butler-Simon N, Rumack CM, Accurso FJ. Role of respiratory syncytial virus in early hospitalizations for respiratory distress of young infants with cystic fibrosis. *J Pediatr* 1988; **113**: 827–30.

7 Wang EL, Prober CG, Manson B, Corey M, Levison H. Association of respiratory viral infections with pulminary deterioration in patients with cystic fibrosis. *N Engl J Med* 1984; **311**: 1653–8.

8 Hordvik NL, König P, Hamory B, *et al.* Effects of acute viral respiratory infections in patients with cystic fibrosis. *Pediatr Pulmonol* 1989; **7**: 217–22.

9 Conway SP, Simmonds EJ, Littlewood JM. Acute severe deterioration in cystic fibrosis associated with influenza-A virus infection. *Thorax* 1992; **47**: 112–4.

10 Johansen HK, Høiby N. Seasonal onset of initial colonisation and chronic infection with Pseudomonas aeruginosa in patients with cystic fibrosis in Denmark. *Thorax* 1992; **47**: 109–11.

11 Shale DJ. Viral infections – a role in the lung disease of cystic fibrosis. *Thorax* 1992; **47**: 69.

12 Høiby N. Microbiology of lung infections in cystic fibrosis patients. *Acta Paediatrica Scandinavica* 1982; **301** (suppl): 33–54.

13 Schønheyder H. Pathogenetic and serological aspects of pulmonary Aspergillosis. *Scand J Infect Dis* 1987; **51** (suppl): 1–62.

14 Forsyth KD, Hohmann AW, Martin AJ, Bradley J. IgG antibodies to aspergillus fumigatus in cystic fibrosis: a laboratory correlate of disease activity. *Arch Dis Child* 1988; **63**: 953–7.

15 Przyklenk B, Bauernfeind A, Hörl G, Emminger G. Serologic response to Candida albicans and Aspergillus fumigatus in cystic fibrosis. *Infection* 1987; **15**: 308–10.

16 Vazquez C, Aramburu N, Sojo A, Vitoria JC, Pascual C. IgG antibodies to Aspergillus fumigatus in cystic fibrosis. *Arch Dis Child* 1989; **64**: 1094–5.

17 Høiby N. Cystic fibrosis: infection. *Schweiz Med Wochenschr* 1991; **121**: 105–9.

18 Govan JRW, Glass S. The microbiology and therapy of cystic fibrosis lung infections. *Rev Med Microbiol* 1990; **1**: 11a–28.

19 Gilligan PH. Microbiology of airway disease in patients with cystic fibrosis. *Clin Microbiol Rev* 1991; **4**: 35–51.

20 Pedersen SS, Jensen T, Pressler T, Høiby N K R Does centralized treatment of

cystic fibrosis increase the risk of Pseudomonas aeruginosa infection? *Acta Paediatrica Scandinavica* 1986; 75: 840–5.

21 Greenberg DP, Stutman HR. Infection and immunity to Staphylococcus aureus and Haemophilus influenzae. *Clin Rev Allergy* 1991; 9: 75–86.

22 Albus A, Fournier J-M, Wolz C, *et al.* Staphylococcus aureus capsular types and antibody response to lung infection in patients with cystic fibrosis. *J Clin Microbiol* 1988; 26: 2505–9.

23 Goering RV, Bauernfeind A, Lenz W, Przyklenk B. Staphylococcus aureus in patients with cystic fibrosis – an epidemiological analysis using a combination of traditional and molecular methods. *Infection* 1990; 18: 57–60.

24 Couetdic G, Estavoyer JM, Fournier JM, Michelbriand Y. Anti-lipoteichoic acid antibodies in 45 cystic fibrosis patients with Staphylococcus aureus infection. *Presse Med* 1991; 20: 1342.

25 Bauernfeind A, Przyklenk B, Matthias C, Jungwirth R, Bertele RM, Harms K. Selection of antibiotics for treatment and prophylaxis of staphylococcal infections in cystic fibrosis patients. *Infection* 1990; 18: 126–30.

26 Jensen T, Pedersen SS, Høiby N, Koch C, Flensborg EW. Use of antibiotics in cystic fibrosis: the Danish approach. In: Høiby N, Pedersen SS, Shand GH, Döring G, Holder IA, eds. *Pseudomonas aeruginosa infection.* Basel: Karger, 1989: 237–46.

27 Marks MI. Antibiotic therapy for bronchopulmonary infections in cystic fibrosis. In: Høiby N, Pedersen SS, Shand GH, Döring G, Holder A, eds. *Pseudomonas aeruginosa infection.* Basel: Karger, 1989: 229–36.

28 Geddes DM. Antimicrobial therapy against Staphylococcus aureus, Pseudomonas aeruginosa, and Pseudomonas cepacia. *Chest* 1988; 94 suppl: 140S–144S.

29 Loening-Baucke VA, Mischler E, Myers MG. A placebo-controlled trial of cephalexin therapy in the ambulatory management of patients with cystic fibrosis. *J Pediat* 1979; 95: 630–7.

30 Nolan G, McIvor P, Levison H, Fleming PC, Corey M, Gold R. Antibiotic prophylaxis in cystic fibrosis: inhaled cephaloridine as an adjunct to oral cloxacillin. *J Pediat* 1982; 101: 626–30.

31 Jensen T, Lang S, Faber M, Rosdahl VT, Høiby N, Koch C. Clinical experiences with fusidic acid in cystic fibrosis patients. *J Antimicrob Chemother* 1990; 25 (suppl B): 45–52.

32 Marks MI. Antibiotic therapy for bronchopulmonary infections in cystic fibrosis. *Chemotherapy* 1989; 42: 229–36.

33 Spino M. Pharmacokinetics of drugs in cystic fibrosis. *Clin Rev Allergy* 1991; 9: 169–210.

34 Mouton JW, Kerrebijn KF. Antibacterial therapy in cystic fibrosis. *Med Clin North Am* 1990; 74: 837–50.

35 Harper JJ, Tilse MH. Biotypes of Haemophilus influenzae that are associated with noninvasive infections. *J Clin Microbiol* 1991; 29: 2539–42.

36 Watson KC, Kerr EJC, Baillie M. Temporal changes in biotypes of Haemophilus influenzae isolated from patients with cystic fibrosis. *J Med Microbiol* 1988; 26: 129–32.

37 Pedersen M, Støvring S, Morkassel E, Koch C, Høiby N. Persistent Haemophilus influenzae infection in the lower respiratory tract of children with chronic lung disease. A comparative study of amoxicillin and pivampicillin. *Scand J Infect Dis* 1986; 18: 245–54.

38 Jensen T, Pedersen SS, Stafanger G, Høiby N, Koch C, Bondesson G. Comparison of amoxycillin/clavulanate (Spektramox) with amoxycillin in children and adults with chronic obstructive pulmonary disease and infection with Haemophilus influenzae. *Scand J Infect Dis* 1988; 20: 517–24.

39 Høiby N, Friis B, Jensen K, *et al.* Antimicrobial chemotherapy in cystic fibrosis patients. *Acta Paediatrica Scandinavica* 1982; 301 (suppl): 75–100.

40 Isles A, Maclusky I, Corey M, *et al.* Pseudomonas cepacia infection in cystic fibrosis: an emerging problem. *J Pediatr* 1984; **104**: 206–10.

41 Baltimore RS, Radnay-Baltimore K, Graevenitz Av, Dolan TF. Occurrence of nonfermentative Gram-negative rods other than Pseudomonas aeruginosa in the respiratory tract of children with cystic fibrosis. *Helv Paediat Acta* 1982; **37**: 547–54.

42 Lewin LO, Byard PJ, Davis PB. Effect of Pseudomonas cepacia colonization on survival and pulmonary function of cystic fibrosis patients. *J Clin Epidemiol* 1990; **43**: 125–31.

43 Laraya-Cuasay LR, Lipstein M, Huang NN. Pseudomonas cepacia in the respiratory flora of patients with cystic fibrosis (CF). *Amer Soc Ped Dis* 1977; 502.

44 Thomassen MJ. Pseudomonas cepacia colonization among patients with cystic fibrosis. *Amer Rev Respir Dis* 1985; **131**: 791–6.

45 Tomashefski JF Jr, Thomassen MJ, Bruce MC, Goldberg HI, Konstan MW, Stern RC. Pseudomonas cepacia-associated pneumonia in cystic fibrosis. *Arch Pathol Lab Med* 1988; **112**: 166–72.

46 Tablan OC, Chorba TL, Schidlow DV, *et al.* Pseudomonas cepacia colonization in patients with cystic fibrosis: risk factors and clinical outcome. *J Pediatr* 1985; **107**: 382–7.

47 Tablan OC, Martone WJ, Doershuk CF, *et al.* Colonization of the respiratory tract with Pseudomonas cepacia in cystic fibrosis. Risk factors and outcomes. *Chest* 1987; **97**: 527–32.

48 Simmonds EJ, Conway SP, Ghoneim ATM, Ross H, Littlewood JM. Pseudomonas cepacia – a new pathogen in patients with cystic fibrosis referred to a large centre in the United Kingdom. *Arch Dis Child* 1990; **65**: 874–7.

49 LiPuma JJ, Mortensen JE, Dasen SE, Edlin TD, Schidlow DV, Burns JL, *et al.* Ribotype analysis of Pseudomonas cepacia from cystic fibrosis treatment centers. *J Pediatr* 1988; **113**: 859–62.

50 Nelson JW, Doherty CJ, Brown PH, Greening AP, Kaufmann ME, Govan JRW. Pseudomonas cepacia in inpatients with cystic fibrosis. *Lancet* 1991; **338**: 1525.

51 Smith DL, Smith EG, Gumery LB, Stableforth DE. Pseudomonas cepacia infection in cystic fibrosis. *Lancet* 1992; **339**: 252.

52 Gladman G, Connor PJ, Williams RF, David TJ. Controlled study of Pseudomonas cepacia and Pseudomonas maltophilia in cystic fibrosis. *Arch Dis Child* 1992; **67**: 192–5.

53 Gessner AR, Mortensen JE. Pathogenic factors of Pseudomonas cepacia isolates from patients with cystic fibrosis. *J Med Microbiol* 1990; **33**: 115–20.

54 Nir M, Johansen HK, Høiby N. Low incidence of pulmonary Pseudomonas cepacia infection in Danish cystic fibrosis patients. *Acta Paediatr* 1992; **81**: 1042–3.

55 Editorial. Pseudomonas cepacia – more than a harmless commensal? *Lancet* 1992; **339**: 1385–6.

56 FitzSimmons SC. The changing epidemiology of cystic fibrosis. *J Pediatr* 1993; **122**: 1–9.

57 Thomassen MJ, Demko CA, Doershuk CF, Stern RC, Klinger JD. Pseudomonas cepacia: decrease in colonization in patients with cystic fibrosis. *Am Rev Respir Dis* 1986; **134**: 669–71.

58 Hardy KA, McGowan KL, Fisher MC, Schidlow DV. Pseudomonas cepacia in the hospital setting: lack of transmission between cystic fibrosis patients. *J Pediatr* 1986; **109**: 51–4.

59 Lipuma JJ, Dasen SE, Nielson DW, Stern RC, Stull TL. Person-to-person transmission of Pseudomonas cepacia between patients with cystic fibrosis. *Lancet* 1990; **336**: 1094–6.

60 Millar-Jones L, Paull A, Saunders Z, Goodchild MC. Transmission of

Pseudomonas cepacia among cystic fibrosis patients. *Lancet* 1992; **340**: 491.

61 Aronoff SC. Outer membrane permeability in pseudomonas cepacia: diminished porin content in a β-lactam-resistant mutant and in resistant cystic fibrosis isolates. *Antimicrob Agents Chemother* 1988; **32**: 1636–9.

62 Kumar A, Wofford-McQueen R, Gordon RC. Ciprofloxacin, imipenem and rifampicin; in-vitro synergy of two and three drug combinations against pseudomonas cepacia. *J Antimicrob Chemother* 1989; **23**: 831–5.

63 Klinger JD, Aronoff SC. In vitro activity of ciprofloxacin and other antibacterial agents against pseudomonas aeruginosa and pseudomonas cepacia from cystic fibrosis patients. *J Antimicrob Chemother* 1985; **15**: 679–84.

64 Bosso JA, Saxon BA, Matsen JM. In vitro activity of aztreonam combined with tobramycin and gentamicin against clinical isolates of pseudomonas aeruginosa and pseudomonas cepacia from patients with cystic fibrosis. *Antimicrob Agents Chemother* 1987; **31**: 1403–5.

65 Cohn RC, Rudzienski L. Observations on amiloride-tobramycin synergy in Pseudomonas cepacia. *Current Therapeutic Research – Clinical and Experimental* 1991; **50**: 786–93.

66 Taylor RFH, Morgan DW, Nicholson PS, Mackay IS, Hodson ME, Pitt TL. Extrapulmonary sites of Pseudomonas aeruginosa in adults with cystic fibrosis. *Thorax* 1992; **47**: 426–8.

67 Agnarsson U, Glass S, Govan JRW. Fecal isolation of Pseudomonas aeruginosa from patients with cystic fibrosis. *J Clin Microbiol* 1989; **27**: 96–8.

68 Speert DP, Campbell ME, Davidson GF, Wong LTK. Pseudomonas aeruginosa colonization of the gastrointestinal tract in patients with cystic fibrosis. *J Infect Dis* 1993; **167**: 226–9.

69 Petersen NT, Høiby N, Mordhorst C-H, Lind K, Flensborg EW, Bruun B. Respiratory infections in cystic fibrosis patients caused by virus, chlamydia and mycoplasma – possible synergism with Pseudomonas aeruginosa. In: Sturgess JM, ed. *Perspectives in cystic fibrosis, proceedings of the 8th international cystic fibrosis congress held in Toronto, Canada May 26–30, 1980.* Toronto: Canadian Cystic Fibrosis Foundation, 1980: 346–51.

70 Kelly NM, Tempany E, Falkner FR, Fitzgerald MX, O'Boyle C, Keane CT. Does Pseudomonas cross-infection occur between cystic fibrosis patients? *Lancet* 1982; **ii**: 688–9.

71 Zimakoff J, Høiby N, Rosendal K, Guilbert JP. Epidemiology of Pseudomonas aeruginosa infection and the role of contamination of the environment in a cystic fibrosis clinic. *J Hosp Infect* 1983; **4**: 31–40.

72 Döring G, Ulrich M, Müller W, *et al.* Generation of Pseudomonas aeruginosa aerosols during handwashing from contaminated sink drains, transmission to hands of hospital personnel, and its prevention by use of a new heating device. *Zentralbl Hyg Umweltmed* 1991; **191**: 494–505.

73 Wolz C, Kiosz G, Ogle JW, *et al.* Pseudomonas aeruginosa cross-colonization and persistence in patients with cystic fibrosis. Use of a DNA probe. *Epidemiol Infect* 1989; **102**: 205–14.

74 Döring G, Bareth H, Gairing A, Wolz C, Botzenhart K. Genotyping of Pseudomonas aeruginosa sputum and stool isolates from cystic fibrosis patients – evidence for intestinal colonization and spreading into toilets. *Epidemiol Infect* 1989; **103**: 555–64.

75 Döring G. Pseudomonas aeruginosa epidemiology: major environmental reservoirs, routes of transmission and strategies for prevention. *Pediatr Pulmonol* 1991; **6** (Suppl): 280.

76 Govan JRW, Nelson JW. Microbiology of lung infection in cystic fibrosis. *Br Med Bull* 1992; **48**: 912–30.

77 Hoogkamp-Korstanje JAA, Laag Jvd. Incidence and risk of cross-colonization in cystic fibrosis holiday camps. *Antonie Van Leeuwenhock* 1980; **46**: 100–1.

78 Speert DP, Lawton D, Damm S. Communicability of Pseudomonas aerugi-

nosa in a cystic fibrosis summer camp. *Clinical and Laboratory Observations* 1982; **101**: 227–9.

78a Høiby N, Pedersen SS. Estimated risk of cross-infection with Pseudomonas aeruginosa in Danish cystic fibrosis patients. *Acta Paediatrica Scandinavica* 1989; **78**: 395–404.

79 Pedersen SS, Koch C, Høiby N, Rosendal K. An epidemic spread of multiresistant Pseudomonas aeruginosa in a cystic fibrosis centre. *J Antimicrob Chemother* 1986; **17**: 505–16.

80 Tummler B, Koopmann U, Grothues D, Weissbrodt H, Steinkamp G, Vonderhardt H. Nosocomial acquisition of Pseudomonas aeruginosa by cystic fibrosis patients. *J Clin Microbiol* 1991; **29**: 1265–7.

81 Speert DP, Campbell ME. Hospital epidemiology of Pseudomonas aeruginosa from patients with cystic fibrosis. *J Hosp Infect* 1987; **9**: 11–21.

82 Pedersen SS. Lung infection with alginate-producing, mucoid Pseudomonas aeruginosa in cystic fibrosis. *APMIS* 1992; **100** (suppl 28): 5–79.

83 Nelson JW, Tredgett MW, Sheehan JK, Thornton DJ, Notman D, Govan JRW. Mucinophilic and chemotactic properties of Pseudomonas aeruginosa in relation to pulmonary colonization in cystic fibrosis. *Infect Immun* 1990; **58**: 1489–95.

84 Baker NR, Svanborg-Edén C. Role of alginate in the adherence of Pseudomonas aeruginosa. In: Høiby N, Pedersen SS, Shand GH, Döring G, Holder IA, eds. *Pseudomonas aeruginosa infection*. Basel: Karger, 1989: 72–9.

85 Ramphal R, Guay C, Pier GB. Pseudomonas aeruginosa adhesins for tracheobronchial mucin. *Infect Immun* 1987; **55**: 600–3.

86 Baker NR, Minor V, Deal C, Shahrabadi MS, Simpson DA, Woods DE. Pseudomonas aeruginosa exoenzyme-S is an adhesin. *Infect Immun* 1991; **59**: 2859–63.

87 Plotkowski MC, Beck G, Tournier JM, Bernardo M, Marques EA, Puchelle E. Adherence of pseudomonas aeruginosa to respiratory epithelium and the effect of leucocyte elastase. *J Med Microbiol* 1989; **30**: 285–93.

88 Döring G, Goldstein W, Röll A, Schiøtz PO, Høiby N, Botzenhart K. The role of Pseudomonas aeruginosa exoenzymes in lung infections of patients with cystic fibrosis. *Infect Immun* 1985; **49**: 557–62.

89 Kharazmi A. Interactions of Pseudomonas aeruginosa proteases with the cells of the immune system. In: Høiby N, Pedersen SS, Shand GH, Döring G, Holder IA, eds. *Pseudomonas aeruginosa infection*. Basel: Karger, 1989: 42–9.

90 Brett MM, Simmonds EJ, Ghoneim ATM, Littlewood JM. The value of serum IgG titres against Pseudomonas aeruginosa in the management of early pseudomonal infection in cystic fibrosis. *Arch Dis Child* 1992; **67**: 1086–8.

91 Döring G, Obernesser H-J, Botzenhart K, Flehmig B, Høiby N, Hofman A. Proteases of Pseudomonas aeruginosa in patients with cystic fibrosis. *J Infect Dis* 1983; **147**: 744–50.

92 Döring G, Høiby N. Longitudinal study of immune response to Pseudomonas aeruginosa antigens in cystic fibrosis. *Infect Immun* 1983; **42**: 197–201.

93 Döring G, Buhl V, Høiby N, Schiøtz PO, Botzenhart K. Detection of proteases of Pseudomonas aeruginosa in immune complexes isolated from sputum of cystic fibrosis patients. *Acta Pathologica et Microbiologica et Immunologia Scandinavica Section C* 1984; **92**: 307–12.

94 Pedersen SS, Høiby N, Espersen F, Koch C. Role of alginate in infection with mucoid Pseudomonas aeruginosa in cystic fibrosis. *Thorax* 1992; **47**: 6–13.

95 Henry RL, Mellis CM, Petrovic L. Mucoid Pseudomonas aeruginosa is a marker of poor survival in cystic fibrosis. *Pediatr Pulmonol* 1992; **12**: 158–61.

96 Baltimore RS, Christie CDC, Smith GJW. Immunohistopathologic localization of pseudomonas aeruginosa in lungs from patients with cystic fibrosis – implications for the pathogenesis of progressive lung deterioration. *Am Rev Resp Dis* 1989; **140**: 1650–61.

97 May TB, Shinabarger D, Maharaj R, *et al*. Alginate synthesis by Pseudomonas aeruginosa – a key pathogenic factor in chronic pulmonary infections in cystic fibrosis patients. *Clin Microbiol Rev* 1991; 4: 191–206.

98 Roychoudhury S, Zielinski NA, Devault JD, *et al*. Pseudomonas aeruginosa infection in cystic fibrosis – biosynthesis of alginate as a virulence factory. *Pseudomonas-Aeruginosa in Human Diseases* 1991; 44: 63–7.

99 Lam J, Chan R, Lam K, Costerton JW. Production of mucoid microcolonies by Pseudomonas aeruginosa within infected lungs in cystic fibrosis. *Infect Immun* 1980; 28: 546–56.

100 Costerton JW, Cheng K-J, Geesey GG, *et al*. Bacterial biofilms in nature and disease. In: Ornston LN, Balows A, Baumann P, eds. *Annual review of microbiology*. Vol 41. Palo Alto: Annual Reviews Inc, 1987: 435–64.

101 Jensen ET, Kharazmi A, Lam K, Costerton JW, Høiby N. Human polymorphonuclear leukocyte response to Pseudomonas aeruginosa grown in biofilm. *Infect Immun* 1990; 58: 2383–5.

102 Høiby N. Prevalence of mucoid strains of Pseudomonas aeruginosa in bacteriological specimens from patients with cystic fibrosis and patients with other diseases. *Acta Pathologica Microbiologica Scandinavica Section B* 1975; 83: 549–52.

103 Anwar H, Dasgupta MK, Costerton JW. Testing the susceptibility of bacteria in biofilms to antibacterial agents. *Antimicrob Agents Chemother* 1990; 34: 2043–6.

104 Anwar H, Strap JL, Costerton JW. Susceptibility of biofilm cells of Pseudomonas aeruginosa to bactericidal actions of whole blood and serum. *FEMS Microbiol Lett* 1992; 92: 235–42.

105 Giwercman B, Lambert PA, Rosdal VT, Shand GH, Høiby N. Rapid emergence of resistance in Pseudomonas aeruginosa in cystic fibrosis patients due to in vivo selection of stable partially derepressed β-lactamase producing strains. *J Antimicrob Chemother* 1990; 26: 247–59.

106 Pedersen SS, Moller H, Espersen F, Sorensen CH, Jensen T, Høiby N. Mucosal immunity to Pseudomonas aeruginosa alginate in cystic fibrosis. *APMIS* 1992; 100: 326–34.

107 Cordon SM, Elborn JS, Rayner RJ, Hiller EJ, Shale DJ. IgG Antibodies in early Pseudomonas aeruginosa infection in cystic fibrosis. *Arch Dis Child* 1992; 67: 737–40.

108 Pier GB, Grout M, Desjardins D. Complement deposition by antibodies to Pseudomonas aeruginosa mucoid exopolysaccharide (MEP) and by non-MEP specific opsonins. *J Immunol* 1991; 147: 1869–76.

109 Penketh ARL, Pitt TL, Hodson ME, Batten JC. Bactericidal activity of serum from cystic fibrosis patients for Pseudomonas aeruginosa. *J Med Microbiol* 1983; 16: 401–8.

110 Ojeniyi B, Høiby N, Rosdal VT. Prevalence and persistence of polyagglutinable Pseudomonas aeruginosa in cystic fibrosis patients. *APMIS* 1991; 99: 187–95.

111 Ojeniyi B, Bæk L, Høiby N. Polyagglutinability due to loss of 0-antigenic determinants in Pseudomonas aeruginosa strains isolated from cystic fibrosis patients. *Acta Pathologica Microbiologica Scandinavica Section B* 1985; 93: 7–13.

112 Shand GH, Pedersen SS, Brown MRW, Høiby N. Serum antibodies to Pseudomonas aeruginosa outer-membrane proteins and iron-regulated membrane proteins at different stages of chronic cystic fibrosis lung infection. *J Med Microbiol* 1991; 34: 203–12.

113 Høiby N, Koch C. Pseudomonas aeruginosa infection in cystic fibrosis and its management. *Thorax* 1990; 45: 881–4.

114 Lam MYC, McGroarty EJ, Kropinski AM, *et al*. The occurrence of a common lipopolysaccharide antigen in standard and clinical strains of Pseudomonas aeruginosa. *J Clin Microbiol* 1989; 27: 962–7.

115 Ojeniyi B, Rosdal VT, Høiby N. Changes in serotype caused by cell to cell contact between different Pseudomonas aeruginosa strains from cystic fibrosis patients. *Acta Pathol Microbiol Scand Sect B* 1987; **95**: 23–7.

116 Ojeniyi B. Bacteriophages in sputum of cystic fibrosis patients as a possible cause of in vivo changes in serotypes of Pseudomonas aeruginosa. *APMIS* 1988; **96**: 294–8.

117 Giwercman B, Fomsgaard A, Mansa B, Høiby N. Polyacrylamide gel electrophoresis analysis of lipopolysaccharide from Pseudomonas aeruginosa growing planctonically and as biofilm. *FEMS Microbiol Immunol* 1992; **89**: 225–30.

118 Kronborg G, Shand GH, Fomsgaard A, Høiby N. Lipopolysaccharide is present in immune complexes isolated from sputum in patients with cystic fibrosis and chronic Pseudomonas aeruginosa lung infection. *APMIS* 1992; **100**: 175–80.

119 Pedersen SS, Høiby N, Shand GH, Pressler T. Antibody response to Pseudomonas aeruginosa antigens in cystic fibrosis. In: Høiby N, Pedersen SS, Shand GH, Döring G, Holder IA, eds. *Pseudomonas aeruginosa infection*. Basel: Karger, 1989: 130–53.

120 Høiby N, Flensborg EW, Beck B, Friis B, Jacobsen L, Vidar Jacobsen S. Pseudomonas aeruginosa infection in cystic fibrosis. Diagnostic and prognostic significance of Pseudomonas aeruginosa precipitins determined by means of crossed immunoelectrophoresis. *Scand J Respir Dis* 1977; **58**: 65–79.

121 Dasgupta MK, Lam J, Döring G, *et al.* Prognostic implications of circulating immune complexes and pseudomonas aeruginosa-specific antibodies in cystic fibrosis. *J Clin Lab Immunol* 1987; **23**: 25–30.

122 Dasgupta MK, Zuberbuhler P, Abbi A, *et al.* Combined evaluation of circulating immune complexes and antibodies to pseudomonas aeruginosa as an immunologic profile in relation to pulmonary function in cystic fibrosis. *J Clin Immunol* 1987; **7**: 51–7.

123 Suter S. The imbalance between granulocyte neutral proteases and anti-proteases in bronchial secretions from patients with cystic fibrosis. In: Høiby N, Pedersen SS, Shand GH, Döring G, Holder IA, eds. *Pseudomonas aeruginosa infection*. Basel: Karger, 1989: 158–68.

124 Goldstein W, Döring G. Lysosomal enzymes from polymorphonuclear leukocytes and proteinase inhibitors in patients with cystic fibrosis. *Am Rev Respir Dis* 1986; **134**: 49–56.

125 Zach MS. Pathogenesis and management of lung disease in cystic fibrosis. *J Roy Soc Med* 1991; **84** (Suppl 18): 10–17.

126 Langford DT, Hiller EJ. Prospective, controlled study of a polyvalent pseudomonas vaccine in cystic fibrosis–three year results. *Arch Dis Child* 1984; **59**: 1131–4.

127 Cryz SJ, Furer E, Que JU, Sadoff JC, Brenner M, Schaad UB. Clinical evaluation of an octavalent Pseudomonas aeruginosa conjugate vaccine in plasma donors and in bone marrow transplant and cystic fibrosis patients. *Pseudomonas-Aeruginosa in Human Diseases* 1991; **44**: 157–62.

128 Schaad UB, Lang AB, Wedgwood J, *et al.* Safety and immunogenicity of Pseudomonas aeruginosa conjugate-A vaccine in cystic fibrosis. *Lancet* 1991; **338**: 1236–7.

129 Pier GB. Vaccine potential of Pseudomonas aeruginosa mucoid exopoly-saccharide (alginate). *Pseudomonas-Aeruginosa in Human Diseases* 1991; **44**: 136–42.

130 Johansen HK, Høiby N, Pedersen SS. Experimental immunization with Pseudomonas aeruginosa alginate induces IgA and IgG antibody responses. *APMIS* 1991; **99**: 1061–8.

131 Johansen HK, Høiby N. Local IgA and IgG response to intratracheal

immunization with Pseudomonas aeruginosa antigens. *APMIS* 1992; **100**: 87–90.

132 Moss RB. Antibody production in CF and possibilities for immunotherapy. *Pediatr Pulmonol* 1990; 5 (Suppl): 66–7.

133 Valerius NH, Koch C, Høiby N. Prevention of chronic Pseudomonas aeruginosa colonisation in cystic fibrosis by early treatment. *Lancet* 1991; **338**: 725–6.

134 Gold R, Carpenter S, Heurter H, Corey M, Levison H. Randomized trial of ceftazidime versus placebo in the management of acute respiratory exacerbations in patients with cystic fibrosis. *Pediatric Pharmacology and Therapeutics* 1987; **111**: 907–13.

135 Kerem E, Corey M, Gold R, Levison H. Pulmonary function and clinical course in patients with cystic fibrosis after pulmonary colonization with Pseudomonas aeruginosa. *J Pediatr* 1990; **116**: 714–9.

136 Regelmann WE, Elliott GR, Warwick WJ, Clawson CC. Reduction of sputum Pseudomonas aeruginosa density by antibiotics improves lung function in cystic fibrosis more than do bronchodilators and chest physiotherapy alone. *Am Rev Respir Dis* 1990; **141**: 914–21.

137 Wood RE, Leigh MW. What is a "pulmonary exacerbation" in cystic fibrosis? *J Pediatr* 1987; **111**: 841–2.

138 Pattishall EA. Negative clinical trials in cystic fibrosis research. *Pediatrics* 1990; **85**: 277–81.

139 Szaff M, Høiby N, Flensborg EW. Frequent antibiotic therapy improves survival of cystic fibrosis patients with chronic Pseudomonas aeruginosa infection. *Acta Paediatrica Scandinavica* 1983; **72**: 651–7.

140 Pedersen SS, Jensen T, Høiby N, Koch C, Flensborg EW. Management of Pseudomonas aeruginosa lung infection in Danish cystic fibrosis patients. *Acta Paediatrica Scandinavica* 1987; **76**: 955–61.

141 Horrevorts AM, White JD, Degener JE, *et al.* Tobramycin in patients with cystic fibrosis: adjustment in dosing interval for effective treatment. *Chest* 1987; **92**: 844–8.

142 Weber A, Degroot R, Ramsey B, Williamswarren J, Smith A. Probenecid pharmacokinetics in cystic fibrosis. *Dev Pharmacol Ther* 1991; **16**: 7–12.

143 Hodson ME, Penketh ARL, Batten JC. Aerosol carbenicillin and gentamicin treatment of pseudomonas aeruginosa infection in patients with cystic fibrosis. *Lancet* 1981; **ii**: 1137–9.

144 Hodson ME, Roberts CM, Butland RJA, Smith MJ, Batten JC. Oral ciprofloxacin compared with conventional intravenous treatment for pseudomonas aeruginosa infection in adults with cystic fibrosis. *Lancet* 1987; **i**: 235–7.

145 Jensen T, Pedersen SS, Høiby N, Koch C. Efficacy of oral fluoroquinolones versus conventional intravenous antipseudomonal chemotherapy in treatment of cystic fibrosis. *Eur J Clin Microbiol* 1988; **6**: 618–22.

146 Moss RB. Drug allergy in cystic fibrosis. *Clin Rev Allergy* 1991; **9**: 211–29.

147 Koch C, Hjelt K, Pedersen SS, *et al.* Retrospective clinical study of hypersensitivity reactions to aztreonam and six other β-lactam antibiotics in cystic fibrosis patients receiving multiple treatment courses. *Rev Infect Dis* 1991; **13** (suppl): S608–11.

148 Jensen T, Pedersen SS, Høiby N, Koch C. Safety of aztreonam in patients with cystic fibrosis and allergy to beta-lactam antibiotics. *Rev Infect Dis* 1991; **13** (suppl): S594–7.

149 Pedersen SS, Pressler T, Jensen T, *et al.* Combined imipenem/cilistatin and tobramycin therapy of multiresistant Pseudomonas aeruginosa in cystic fibrosis. *J Antimicrob Chemother* 1987; **19**: 101–7.

150 Jensen T, Pedersen SS, Nielsen CH, Høiby N, Koch C. Comparison of the efficacy and safety of ciprofloxacin and ofloxacin in the treatment of chronic

Pseudomonas aeruginosa infection in cystic fibrosis patients. *J Antimicrob Chemother* 1987; **20**: 585–94.

151 Giwercman B, Meyer C, Lambert PA, Reinert C, Høiby N. High-level beta-lactamase activity in sputum samples from cystic fibrosis patients during antipseudomonal treatment. *Antimicrob Agents Chemother* 1992; **36**: 71–6.

152 Dostal RE, Seale JP, Yan BJ. Resistance to ciprofloxacin of respiratory pathogens in patients with cystic fibrosis. *Med J Aust* 1992; **156**: 20–4.

153 Pedersen SS, Jensen T, Osterhammel D, Osterhammel P. Cumulative and acute toxicity of repeated high-dose tobramycin treatment in cystic fibrosis. *Antimicrob Agents Chemother* 1987; **31**: 594–9.

154 Collins MT, McDonald J, Høiby N, Aalund O. Agglutinating antibody titres to Legionellaceae in cystic fibrosis patients as a result of cross-reacting antibodies to Pseudomonas aeruginosa. *J Clin Microbiol* 1984; **19**: 757–62.

155 Hjelte L, Petrini B, Kallenius G, Strandvik B. Prospective study of mycobacterial infections in patients with cystic fibrosis. *Thorax* 1990; **45**: 397–400.

156 Boxerbaum B. Isolation of rapidly growing mycobacteria in patients with cystic fibrosis. *J Pediatr* 1980; **96**: 689–191.

157 Smith MJ, Efthimiou J, Hodson M, Batten JC. Mycobacterial isolations in young adults with cystic fibrosis. *Thorax* 1984; **39**: 369–75.

158 Mulherin D, Coffey MJ, Halloran DO, Keogan MT, Fitzgerald MX. Skin reactivity to atypical mycobacteria in cystic fibrosis. *Respir Med* 1990; **84**: 273–6.

159 Kilby JM, Gilligan PH, Yankaskas JR, Highsmith WE, Edwards LJ, Knowles MR. Nontuberculous mycobacteria in adult patients with cystic fibrosis. *Chest* 1992; **102**: 70–5.

160 Efthimiou J, Smith MJ, Hodson ME, Batten JC. Fatal pulmonary infection with mycobacterium fortuitum in cystic fibrosis. *Br J Dis Chest* 1984; **78**: 299–302.

161 Mearns M, Longbottom J, Batten J. Precipitating antibodies to Aspergillus fumigatus in cystic fibrosis. *Lancet* 1967; **i**: 538–9.

162 Knutsen AP, Slavin RG. Allergic bronchopulmonary aspergillosis in patients with cystic fibrosis. *Clin Rev Allergy* 1991; **9**: 103–18.

163 Carswell F, Hamilton A. Pathogenesis and management of aspergillosis in cystic fibrosis. *Arch Dis Child* 1990; **65**: 1288.

164 Edwards JH, Alfaham M, Fifield R, Philpot C, Clement MJ, Goodchild MC. Sequential serological responses to Aspergillus fumigatus in patients with cystic fibrosis – use of antigen stretching to delineate IgG and IgE activity. *Clin Exp Immunol* 1990; **81**: 101–8.

165 Knutsen AP, Hutcheson PS, Mueller KR, Slavin RG. Serum immunoglobulin-E and immunoglobulin-G anti-Aspergillus fumigatus antibody in patients with cystic fibrosis who have allergic bronchopulmonary aspergillosis. *J Lab Clin Med* 1990; **116**: 724–7.

166 Hutcheson PS, Rejent AJ, Slavin RG. Variability in parameters of allergic bronchopulmonary aspergillosis in patients with cystic fibrosis. *J Allerg Clin Immunol* 1991; **88**: 390–4.

167 Hiller EJ. Pathogenesis and management of aspergillosis in cystic fibrosis. *Arch Dis Child* 1990; **65**: 397–8.

168 Maguire S, Moriarty P, Tempany E, FitzGerald M. Unusual clustering of allergic bronchopulmonary aspergillosis in children with cystic fibrosis. *J Pediatr* 1988; **82**: 835–9.

169 Pinel C, Grillot R, Gout JP, Lebeau B, Bost M, Ambroisethomas P. Cystic fibrosis and allergic bronchopulmonary aspergillosis. *Pathol Biol* 1991; **39**: 617–20.

170 Simmonds EJ, Littlewood JM, Evans EGV. Cystic fibrosis and allergic bronchopulmonary aspergillosis. *Arch Dis Child* 1990; **65**: 507–11.

171 Denning DW, Vanwye JE, Lewiston NJ, Stevens DA. Adjunctive therapy of allergic bronchopulmonary aspergillosis with itraconazole. *Chest* 1991; **100**: 813–9.

172 Orenstein DM, Pattishall EN, Nixon PA, Ross EA, Kaplan RM. Quality of well-being before and after antibiotic treatment of pulmonary exacerbation in patients with cystic fibrosis. *Chest* 1990; **98**: 1081–4.

7 Gastrointestinal and nutritional aspects

HINDA KOPELMAN

Cystic fibrosis is the most common lethal genetic disorder among white people, and the main cause of pancreatic insufficiency and chronic lung disease in childhood. Though most cases are diagnosed in childhood, advances in the diagnosis and treatment during the past two decades have increased the median survival to 28–31 years.[1,2] In a recent survey of people with cystic fibrosis in the United States, a third had reached adulthood in 1990,[2] which is consistent with the expectation that cystic fibrosis will be encountered more often by physicians who look after adults. The incidence of many of the gastrointestinal complications has increased with age, which emphasises the importance of these problems in the care of adult patients.[2] In addition, cystic fibrosis is a major cause of refractory malnutrition in older patients and new approaches to nutritional management and intervention are increasingly important in their overall care. In this chapter I will review the pancreatic, intestinal, hepatobiliary, and nutritional disturbances that are characteristic of cystic fibrosis and some of the current developments in our understanding of their pathogenesis, and our approaches to management.

Pathogenesis

During the 1980s two important findings changed our understanding of cystic fibrosis. The first group of observations led to recognition that certain epithelial chloride channels and their regulation are defective in tissues that express the cystic fibrosis phenotype,[34] and the second was the identification, cloning and sequencing of the cystic fibrosis gene on the long arm of chromosome 7.[5] The cystic fibrosis gene product, cystic fibrosis transmembrane conductance regulator (CFTR), is a large membrane-spanning protein that functions as an epithelial chloride channel.[6] CFTR may have other functions that have yet to be clarified, but abnormal regulation of epithelial chloride ion transport can account for the experimental findings in a number of tissues classically affected in the disease (Figure 7.1). Chloride impermeability in the sweat ducts of patients with cystic fibrosis gives rise to the well known finding of raised chloride concentration in sweat, the standard diagnostic test for cystic fibrosis. Exocrine glands that depend on the epithelial transport of anions to move water across membranes and into secretions may become obstructed as a result of macromolecular hyperconcentration, which leads to difficulties in the clearance of these secretions. Study of pancreatic secretions in cystic fibrosis, well-controlled for

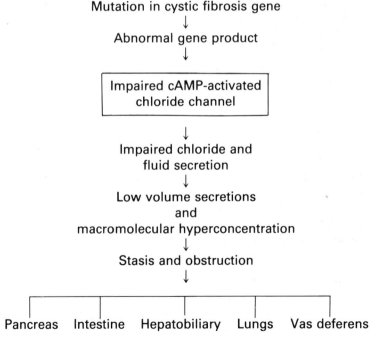

Figure 7.1 The pathogenesis and clinical manifestations of cystic fibrosis.

103

Gastrointestinal manifestations of cystic fibrosis

Pancreatic:	Relative incidence (%)
Insufficiency	80–85
Sufficiency	15–20
Pancreatitis	2–3
Abnormal glucose tolerance	30–50
Diabetes mellitus	1–13
Intestinal:	
Meconium ileus	10–15
Atresias	Not known
Rectal prolapse	20
Distal obstruction syndrome	10–20
Hepatobiliary:	
Cholestasis in infancy	Not known
Fatty liver	15–40
Focal biliary fibrosis	11–70
Multilobular cirrhosis	2–5
Abnormalities of the gallbladder	45
Cholelithiasis	4–12
Obstruction of the common bile duct	Not known

---

pancreatic dysfunction, provides strong evidence in support of this hypothesis.[7]

Pancreatic manifestations

The earliest characteristic morphological feature of the pancreas in cystic fibrosis is the accumulation of secretory material within ducts that is associated with ductal obstruction. Subsequent tissue damage, presumably from acinar release of lytic enzymes, leads to the progressive loss of functioning acinar tissue, fibrosis, and fatty replacement which are the hallmarks of the pancreatic lesion in cystic fibrosis.

The degree of pancreatic tissue destruction in cystic fibrosis is highly variable, which accounts for the differences in clinical presentation and severity of pancreatic manifestations (Box). The main determinant of the severity of pancreatic involvement is the cystic fibrosis genotype, or specific genetic mutation in CFTR. Well over 400 distinct mutations have been identified, some of which confer a mild phenotype, and others a more severe presentation.

The commonest mutation, F508, when it occurs in homozygous presentation, confers a severe form of pancreatic involvement.

Pancreatic insufficiency

Roughly 85% of patients with cystic fibrosis have such severe loss of pancreatic acinar tissue that inadequate secretion of digestive enzymes causes malabsorption. Clinically these people present with large, bulky, greasy stools and poor weight gain or frank weight loss. They may develop signs of fat soluble vitamin deficiencies. Taurine, bile salts, and essential fatty acid deficiencies secondary to malabsorption may contribute to the pathophysiology, and indicate a poor long term prognosis.

Pancreatic insufficiency in cystic fibrosis can be diagnosed by an assessment of fat absorption or of the patient's ability to degrade specific markers such as bentiromide or fluorescein dilaurate.[8] The assessment of fat absorption remains the gold standard and requires a minimum 72 hour fat balance study to assess stool fat output as a percentage of dietary fat intake. Direct assessment of the secretory capacity of the pancreas, though far more invasive and difficult to do, offers the advantage of increased sensitivity. Using this latter approach, patients with pancreatic insufficiency have been shown to retain less than 2% of the normal secretory capacity of the pancreas.[8 9] Activities of pancreatic enzymes in serum, such as pancreatic serum trypsinogen, may be helpful in diagnosing pancreatic insufficiency in some patients with cystic fibrosis. Trypsinogen activity is increased in patients with cystic fibrosis at birth, and is the basis for neonatal screening programmes for cystic fibrosis, but it declines to abnormally low values in patients with pancreatic insufficiency as pancreatic acinar tissue is largely replaced by fibrosis and fat. Empirically this occurs in children over 7–8 years old, making this relatively simple diagnostic test useful for screening adults with cystic fibrosis for pancreatic function.

Successful management of pancreatic insufficiency can usually be achieved by supplementation with commercial preparations of pancreatic enzymes. Enteric-coated enzyme preparations are more effective and require fewer pills because they avoid inactivation by gastric acid. These preparations have virtually replaced the use of capsules containing powdered pancreatic extract. For infants, recommendations of one capsule of a non-microsphere-coated preparation/four ounces of infant formula has often been the initiation dose, with adjustments made as necessary. The enzyme

105

should not be added to the formula but rather mixed in a few teaspoons of strained food. For older children and adults, acid resistant microsphere preparations are recommended because of their improved efficiency. One guideline has been one capsule containing 4000 units of lipase/kg body weight/day to a maximum of 30 capsules/day. These should be given divided into three meals/day and as many snacks as are consumed. It is clear that the variability in dietary intake, pancreatic residual capacity, and pancreatic enzyme release and activation, necessitate an individualised approach to pancreatic enzyme replacement. The actual dose of enzyme must be adjusted considering the number and type of stools and more importantly weight gain and growth.

It is important to remember that not all patients will normalise stool fat excretion by taking pancreatic enzymes. Provided weight, growth, and nutritional status are within normal limits, loss of fat in stools can be tolerated. When in a small number of cases uncorrected malabsorption adversely affects nutritional state despite appropriate pancreatic enzyme replacement, consideration may be given to the pharmacological suppression of gastric acid secretion to improve pancreatic enzyme uncoating, release, and activation. This may be achieved by giving either H_2 antagonists or the prostaglandin analogue misoprostil.[10] It has been suggested that increased gastric acid secretion in cystic fibrosis[11] or decreased bicarbonate secretion[12] or both, with consequent inadequate alkalinisation of the intestinal milieu, adversely affects release and activation of enzymes. High dose enteric-coated pancreatic enzymes with two to four times the enzyme content/capsule of the original preparations are now available and provide the advantage to patients of fewer pills/meal. These preparations should be used under supervision to ensure optimal but not excessive dosing, to contain costs and to reduce potential long term problems; they have been associated with colonic strictures and their use in children is currently being questioned (Chapter 1).

Pancreatic sufficiency

Roughly 15%–20% of patients with cystic fibrosis retain sufficient functional acinar tissue to digest and absorb nutrients normally and do not require pancreatic enzyme supplementation. They are an extremely interesting group who have a better overall prognosis than their counterparts with pancreatic insufficiency[13] and do not usually develop some of the other gastrointestinal complications of cystic fibrosis, such as hepatobiliary disease and the distal intestinal obstruction syndrome. These patients are usually not homozygous for the commonest abnormal cystic fibrosis allele, the F508 deletion.[5] None the less, they do have many of the characteristic clinical findings of cystic fibrosis, particularly defective fluid and chloride secretion and abnormal anion transport. Because of their more limited disease, they have allowed us to learn a great deal about the primary pathophysiology of the pancreatic lesion in cystic fibrosis.

Normal fat digestion on three day fat balance studies or normal bentiromide or fluorescein dilaurate testing identify patients with pancreatic sufficiency, but these tests are not sensitive enough to be of further value. Using duodenal intubation, a marker perfusion technique, and a standard exogenous intravenous pancreatic stimulus, it has been possible to assess pancreatic function quantitatively and accurately. This has shown that there is a tremendous pancreatic reserve and a variability in residual pancreatic exocrine capacity in these patients, ranging from 2%–100% of normal enzyme secretory capacity[8 9] Despite the preservation of normal or near normal enzyme secretory capacity in some patients, their ability to secrete fluid was defective compared with controls with equivalent pancreatic function, accounting for increased concentrations of proteins and poor clearance of secretions.[7] The defect in fluid secretion was caused by diminished secretion of both chloride and bicarbonate ions[12] consistent with the abnormal epithelial anion transport seen in other cystic fibrosis tissues.[3,4]

It is becoming clear that some of these patients with pancreatic sufficiency have progressive destruction of exocrine tissue and loss of function,[14] presumably from continuing or recurrent ductal obstruction, and they may eventually require enzyme supplements. The likelihood of developing insufficiency may be related to the patient's own degree of pancreatic reserve. Quantitative testing may be a useful prognostic tool indicating the residual pancreatic function capacity and the likelihood of destroying that reserve with time.

Pancreatitis

Among the group of patients with cystic fibrosis and pancreatic sufficiency, recurrent pancreatitis may be a problem as it affects 10%–15% of them. These patients have sufficient surviving exocrine tissue to be affected by ductal obstruction and acinar release of enzymes. Because they often have a milder clinical course without many of the other hallmarks of cystic fibrosis, and may not be diagnosed as having cystic fibrosis, recurrent pancreatitis should be an indication for sweat testing.

Diabetes mellitus

At least 30%–50% of patients with cystic fibrosis and pancreatic insufficiency will have abnormal glucose tolerance. It is thought that progressive pancreatic fibrosis ultimately disrupts the function of pancreatic islet cells. Frank diabetes mellitus is less common, occurring in 1%–13% of patients depending on age, and tends to occur later in the course of the disease. Its clinical presentation is the result of insulinopenia and often requires treatment with insulin.

Intestinal manifestations

The main manifestations are the result of partial or complete obstruction of the lumen of the intestinal tract. Obstruction can occur in the uterus, presenting at birth, or at any time during postnatal life. Intestinal presentations of cystic fibrosis (all of which are indications for sweat testing), include meconium ileus, meconium peritonitis, intestinal atresias, unexplained intestinal obstruction, and rectal prolapse.

Meconium ileus

The earliest indication of cystic fibrosis, occurring in 10%–15% of patients, may present in utero with polyhydramnios, or within 48 hours of birth as a small intestinal obstruction with thick inspissated meconium, or both. Classically the newborn infant fails to pass meconium and develops progressive abdominal distension and bilious vomiting. Abdominal radiographs show distended loops of small bowel, absent or scarce air-fluid levels, and bubbles of gas and stool trapped throughout the small bowel. Barium enema examination shows an unused "microcolon." If complicated by intestinal perforation in the uterus, meconium peritonitis results that is associated with ascites, adhesions, and intra-abdominal calcification evident in the radiograph. Other associated intestinal complications include intestinal volvulus, and jejunal and ileal atresias. While none of these findings are pathognomonic of cystic fibrosis, all are strong indications for sweat testing because most infants with meconium ileus, with or without peritonitis, and 15%–20% with intestinal atresias, will have cystic fibrosis.

In uncomplicated meconium ileus, non-surgical relief of

obstruction may be achieved with water-soluble hypertonic enemas (meglumine (Gastrografin) or sodium (Hypaque) diatizoate) given under fluoroscopic control. This is contraindicated in the presence of perforation, peritonitis, or evidence suggestive of volvulus or atresia. In these cases, or if non-surgical manoeuvres fail, operation is essential. With the improvement of surgical management, nutritional support, and postoperative care, mortality is low and the prognosis of infants with meconium ileus, once past the neonatal period, is no different from that of other patients with cystic fibrosis.

Distal intestinal obstruction syndrome

The distal intestinal obstruction syndrome, or "meconium ileus equivalent," includes a range of clinical conditions that result from partial or complete intestinal obstruction after the neonatal period. The pathophysiology probably involves inspissation of intestinal secretions secondary to a combination of pancreatic insufficiency with diminished proteolytic degradation of mucoproteinaceous secretions, and poor clearance of hyperconcentrated dehydrated mucin and intestinal contents. Intestinal mucosal epithelial cells possess defects in chloride and fluid transport[15-18] similar to those seen in other cystic fibrosis epithelial cells. In addition, it has been proposed that disordered intestinal motility with delayed transit may further contribute to the occurrence of this condition.[19]

The clinical presentation is highly variable ranging from recurrent crampy abdominal pain with or without an asymptomatic palpable right lower quadrant mass to complete intestinal obstruction with abdominal distension, tenderness, and vomiting. It is often difficult to differentiate from the far less common conditions that require operation such as appendicitis, appendiceal abscess, intussusception, and caecal neoplasm. The presence of large amounts of faecal material in the right lower quadrant on abdominal radiograph, Gastrografin enema examination, abdominal ultrasound scan, or computed tomogram, and resolution with treatment of the obstruction may all be of diagnostic help.

Operation is rarely required. Medical management has traditionally consisted of increased amounts of pancreatic enzyme replacement; stool softeners such as mineral oil, psyllium hydrophilic mucilloid, and fibre; Gastrografin and other enemas; and in the past, N-acetyl cysteine given orally or rectally. In the absence of complete intestinal obstruction, balanced isotonic electrolyte solutions for gastrointestinal lavage have more recently been given

109

orally or by nasogastric infusion with excellent results.[20] Prokinetic agents such as cisapride may have a role in the prevention of recurrent symptoms in some patients but have not been shown to be useful as an alternative to lavage for the alleviation of partial obstruction.

Constipation

Patients with cystic fibrosis may develop constipation; this may be a sign of the distal intestinal obstruction syndrome or simply a symptom as seen commonly in the general population. Unfortunately the tendency to manage it by reducing the dose of pancreatic enzymes induces malabsorption of fat. This may alleviate the constipation but the price is loss of energy and fat soluble vitamin and nutrient intake. In addition, enzyme reduction may sometimes precipitate an episode of distal intestinal obstruction. We and others have therefore encouraged the treatment of "constipation" in patients with cystic fibrosis with stool softeners rather than reducing their enzyme supplements, with success.

Rectal prolapse

Rectal prolapse occurs in about 20% of patients and may be the first sign of the disease. It is usually recurrent in the first few years of life, spontaneously resolves by 5 years of age, and often improves once treatment for pancreatic insufficiency has begun. It rarely requires operation, although this may be indicated if there is serious pain or incontinence. Rectal prolapse may also occur in cystic fibrosis in the absence of pancreatic insufficiency. Under these circumstances, attempts to reduce constipation or straining during bowel movements may be of benefit.

Other gastrointestinal problems

Patients with cystic fibrosis have other gastrointestinal problems which may or may not be related to cystic fibrosis. They can develop appendicitis and appendiceal abscesses. Failure to respond to treatment for distal intestinal obstruction should alert clinicians to this possibility. The other condition often confused with distal intestinal obstruction syndrome is intestinal intussusception which occurs in patients with cystic fibrosis at an older age than in children. If suspected, a barium or Gastrografin enema examination can be both diagnostic and therapeutic. Operation should be reserved for complications or failure of radiological intervention.

Gastro-oesophageal reflux is extremely common, as is oesophagitis and peptic ulcer disease. These should be managed with aggressive medical intervention as they may result in important morbidity, including adverse effects on nutritional state. Operation is rarely required and should be reserved for complications such as oesophageal stricture, Barrett's oesophagus, or perforated peptic ulcer. There have also been reports of coeliac disease and Crohn's disease in patients with cystic fibrosis.

Pathological, radiological, and functional abnormalities

Findings in the intestinal mucosa that are sufficiently characteristic to be diagnostic of cystic fibrosis include increased numbers of mucin-filled goblet cells, dilated mucin-filled crypts, and eosinophilic casts. Common radiological findings include thickened duodenal folds, nodular filling defects, and variable dilatation of intestinal loops. These findings probably have little clinical importance and should not be interpreted as signs of "duodenitis," ulceration, or inflammatory or infiltrative disease without further confirmation.

Selective intestinal absorption defects in amino acids and bile acids have been reported in cystic fibrosis. These remain to be confirmed and further elucidated, but, clinically important defects in intestinal mucosal structure and function are not evident. Villous structure is intact, D-xylose absorption is within normal limits, and intestinal lactase activity is either within normal limits or even raised in patients with cystic fibrosis. If lactose intolerance occurs it reflects the normal ethnic and age-related incidence in the population and is unrelated to cystic fibrosis.

Hepatobiliary manifestations

The incidence of hepatobiliary manifestations in cystic fibrosis is shown in the box. The more common abnormalities have little effect on overall health and wellbeing and include obstructive jaundice in infancy, which is probably secondary to bile plugs, and often resolves; it is not necessarily associated with liver disease later in life, although this is not entirely clear. Hepatomegaly is caused by fatty changes which may be present even without appreciable malnutrition and may therefore reflect some underlying abnormality in lipid metabolism, oxidative stress, or other metabolic derangement secondary to the cystic fibrosis defect; perhaps it is an early sign of serious cystic fibrosis liver disease. A non-functioning or microgallbladder may not be associated with clinical symptoms.

Focal biliary fibrosis

The characteristic histological lesion in the liver in cystic fibrosis is focal biliary fibrosis, which occurs in patients who are free of symptoms and often in the absence of biochemical evidence of liver disease. Necropsy studies have clearly shown the increasing incidence with age: 11% in infants, 27% in 1 year olds, and 70% in adults. It is characterised by inspissated eosinophilic material in dilated ductules, bile duct proliferation, periductular cell infiltrates, and variable fibrosis and is probably the hepatobiliary variant of the obstructive pathophysiology seen in cystic fibrosis.

A primary abnormality in hepatobiliary anion transport was suggested by evidence that patients with cystic fibrosis regardless of their pancreatic state, have significantly lower concentrations of bile salts in the bile than controls without cystic fibrosis.[21] This might result in diminished bile flow, stasis, and obstruction in the biliary tree. Recently a primary defect in biliary chloride transport was strongly supported by a number of investigations. The expression of the CFTR messenger RNA and protein in normal intrahepatic and extrahepatic biliary epithelium as well as in gallbladder epithelium has been clearly shown by *in situ* hybridisation and immunohistochemistry.[22] Epithelial chloride channels have been found in these tissues which behave like the normal CFTR channel, but which are defective in patients with cystic fibrosis.[23]

Multilobular biliary cirrhosis

Multilobular cirrhosis with hepatosplenomegaly and portal hypertension is an important problem in cystic fibrosis. While cirrhosis in cystic fibrosis rarely causes hepatocellular failure in children, it does occur in association with portal hypertension and oesophageal varices in 2%–5% of adult patients. Because parenchymal liver cells are often spared, hepatocellular function is usually within normal limits, or with only mildly raised liver enzyme activities, bilirubin concentration, and altered measures of coagulation. Despite this, hepatosplenomegaly is quite prominent and is usually the presenting feature. The edge of the liver is firm to hard and nodular. These patients often develop problems associated with portal hypertension, including oesophageal variceal bleeding and hypersplenism.

The pathogenesis remains controversial. To date no association has been shown between the development of liver disease and any specific genotype in cystic fibrosis. Multilobular cirrhosis may be the result of silent progression of the lesion of focal biliary fibrosis. It has also been proposed that stenosis of the common bile duct secondary to pancreatic fibrosis, and intrahepatic biliary tract abnormalities similar to sclerosing cholangitis (both reported in patients with cystic fibrosis) may be responsible for the development of the multilobular cirrhosis seen in cystic fibrosis.[24 25] Though common bile duct stenosis has been clearly shown in patients with cystic fibrosis, the prevalence of this lesion in all patients with cystic fibrosis and liver disease has been questioned and remains to be confirmed. The beading and stricturing of both intrahepatic and extrahepatic ducts which resembles sclerosing cholangitis could result from the accumulation and adherence of mucus and protein in the ducts rather than be a true sclerosing cholangitic lesion.

The diagnosis of liver disease in cystic fibrosis is problematical and possibly the most useful diagnostic variable is physical examination of the patient for an enlarged liver or spleen. Liver enzyme activities are only mildly raised, ultrasonography may confirm the presence of an echogenic liver and enlargement of liver or spleen, or both, and percutaneous liver biopsy has been shown to be unreliable and misleading in view of the patchy nature of the cystic fibrosis lesion. Nuclide scans to assess biliary excretion may be of some value.

The management of hepatic failure, portal hypertension, hypersplenism, ascites, and variceal bleeding in cystic fibrosis does not differ from the recommended treatment of these disorders in general. Sclerotherapy of oesophageal variceal bleeding[26] and hepatic transplantation have both been successfully accomplished in patients with cystic fibrosis. Recently the use of transcutaneous intrahepatic portal shunting has been reported to be useful in cystic fibrosis as a relatively non-invasive measure to reduce the portal hypertension and the incidence of variceal bleeding in patients in whom sclerotherapy fails. The long term efficacy of this procedure is still questioned, but it may offer a relatively benign therapeutic temporising measure before consideration of transplantation or other operation that requires general anaesthesia.

Unfortunately, no treatment is currently available to retard or reverse the process of biliary injury in cystic fibrosis. Experimental approaches including supplementation with taurine, or ursodeoxy-

113

cholic acid or both, have been and are being tried to minimise putative toxic effects as well as enhance bile flow. Recently studies from Europe have shown that oral supplementation with urso-deoxycholic acid in patients with liver disease led to reductions in liver enzyme activities[27 28] and improvement in bile flow as documented by diisopropyl iminodiacetic acid (DISIDA) nuclear scanning of biliary excretion.[29] Questions still remain about the long term effects of this treatment, both beneficial and adverse, in cystic fibrosis; its role in established cirrhosis compared with prevention of this complication; the patients to whom this "prophylaxis" should be given because high risk groups have not yet been clearly identified; and the efficacy of the approach.

The longevity of patients with cystic fibrosis has increased appreciably during the past 30 years. Mean survival in the United States has been reported as 28 years and in Canada as 31 years and between a quarter and a third of patients in the United States were adults. While the prevalence of cirrhosis with portal hypertension in these patients was relatively constant in different age groups over the age of 6 years, the increase in survival suggests that the prevalence of this form of liver disease will increase leading to increased morbidity.

Biliary stones

Intrahepatic and extrahepatic biliary stones are another clinically relevant hepatobiliary problem in cystic fibrosis. Their occurrence may be related to the excessive intestinal loss of bile salts in patients with cystic fibrosis and pancreatic insufficiency, and their tendency to produce lithogenic bile. Alternatively, abnormalities of bile salt, anion, and fluid secretion may predispose to stone formation. Symptomatic cholelithiasis should be managed as generally recommended. The advent of laparoscopic cholecystectomy may result in a reduction in the morbidity associated with the traditional surgical approach.

Nutritional manifestations

Patients with cystic fibrosis are at risk of nutritional deficiencies as a result of three major problems (Figure 7.2). Firstly, malabsorption which leads to excessive loss of macronutrients, energy, and micronutrients such as vitamins, minerals, and bile salts. Secondly, increased requirements as a result of the increased energy expenditure that is related to chronic lung disease,

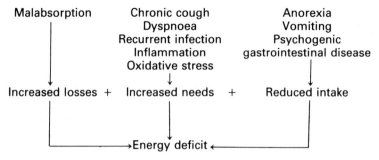

Figure 7.2   Pathogenesis of malnutrition in cystic fibrosis.

continuous inflammation, acute exacerbations of infection, and metabolic derangements including diabetes mellitus. Thirdly, reduced intakes as a result of pulmonary disease; anorexia and vomiting; gastrointestinal complications such as oesophagitis, gastro-oesophageal reflux, distal intestinal obstruction, and biliary tract disease; depression and behavioural problems; and iatrogenic dietary restrictions in energy resulting from recommendations of a low fat diet. While energy expenditure was initially reported to be increased in cystic fibrosis secondary to a basic cellular defect related to the cystic fibrosis gene,[30] subsequent studies that were controlled for both pulmonary function and genotype have not supported this. All three factors contribute to the common development of both macronutrient and micronutrient deficiencies, which may be severe. Insufficient intake of energy and nutrients to meet requirements accounts for the features of protein energy malnutrition which presents as failure to thrive or hypoalbuminaemia and oedema in infancy; poor weight gain and growth; pubertal developmental delay; muscle wasting; and vitamin, mineral, and essential fatty acid deficiencies.

Standard management of malabsorption includes pancreatic enzyme and fat soluble vitamin supplementation. Pancreatic enzyme replacement is somewhat empirical because of the variability in dietary consumption, pancreatic reserve and, intestinal milieu. Vitamin supplementation in patients with cystic fibrosis with pancreatic insufficiency is almost always necessary to meet requirements for fat soluble vitamins. Usually, a multivitamin preparation containing A and D is prescribed at twice the daily requirement for age (vitamin A—8000 IU; vitamin D—800 IU), with 100–200 IU of vitamin E. Vitamin K, 5 mg twice weekly may be prescribed routinely or as necessary. Monitoring of vitamin

115

concentrations (A, E, D, and K) may help to assess the need for increased or decreased supplementation and the degree of compliance with recommendations.

Most cystic fibrosis clinics now recommend and actively encourage consumption of high-energy, balanced diets instead of low fat diets, which tended to limit energy and essential fatty acid consumption. Encouragement of large portions, second helpings, and provision of high energy snacks between meals should be promoted from early childhood. Oral liquid energy supplements may be recommended to help patients meet their increased energy requirements which have been estimated to be about 120%–150% of the required nutrient intakes for age.

When growth and weight gain are not optimal, assessments of dietary intake at home, compliance with pancreatic supplementary enzymes, and 72 hour faecal fat excretion as a percentage of dietary fat intake are essential. Malabsorption should be minimised and energy intake maximised. Gastrointestinal complications that interfere with intake or absorption should be considered, and psychosocial issues that interfere with optimal compliance and management should be dealt with as directly as possible. Pulmonary function should be reassessed and lung disease managed aggressively. Unfortunately, as the disease progresses, a proportion of patients become increasingly more malnourished as their intakes fail to meet requirements despite intensive dietary counselling and encouragement. Under these circumstances, more aggressive approaches to nutritional rehabilitation have been proposed and are generally accepted, including the use of total parenteral nutrition,[31 32] and nocturnal enteral feeding of high energy formulas through a nasogastric tube,[33] or by gastrostomy[34] or jejunostomy[35] infusions. Nasogastric feeding requires a sustained commitment from the patient for nightly insertion of the tube and removal the following morning, and may be hampered by the presence of nasal polyps and congestion, as well as frequent regurgitation of the tube with a severe chronic cough. Interestingly, despite the high incidence of occult gastro-oesophageal reflux in cystic fibrosis, nasogastric tube feeding is usually well tolerated. Surgical placement of jejunostomy tubes has been successful in avoiding problems with gastro-oesophageal reflux. Some centres have concentrated on the use of percutaneous gastrostomy tubes and buttons, which do not require a general anaesthetic or laparotomy and cause little difficulty with reflux. The head of the patient's bed should be raised during feeds, which should be completed at least 1–2 hours before physiotherapy or removal of the nasogastric tube. Prokinetic agents such as domperidone or cisapride may be used to stimulate gastric emptying. The provision of an additional 1000–2000 calories/night using elemental, semi-elemental, and polymeric products by any of these routes has been successful in achieving improved weight gain. Unless a polymeric formulation is used, pancreatic enzyme supplementation is not required with these feeds.

All patients given supplemental feeding gain weight and height, provided that both compliance and management are optimal. In addition to weight gain, growth, and pubertal development, the improvement in nutritional state should on theoretical grounds increase respiratory muscle strength and immunity and may therefore have important long term effects on pulmonary state and survival. Retrospective cross-sectional studies have shown a correlation between nutritional state, improved pulmonary state,[1 13] and overall survival figures.[1] Nocturnal feeding and improved nutritional state have been reported to be associated with improved wellbeing, slower deterioration of pulmonary function,[34 35] and a tendency to improve expiratory respiratory muscle strength.[36] With the advent of lung transplantation, the need to maintain and improve nutritional state to optimise the surgical and postoperative course has increased. The prospect of gene therapy to cure or prevent the pulmonary manifestations of cystic fibrosis strengthens the argument for maintaining an optimal state in patients with cystic fibrosis who may one day benefit from this approach.

References

1 Corey M, McLaughlin FJ, Williams M, Levison H. A comparison of survival, growth, and pulmonary function in patients with cystic fibrosis in Boston and Toronto. *J Clin Epidemiol* 1988; 41: 583–91.
2 FitzSimmons S. The changing epidemiology of cystic fibrosis. *J Pediatr* 1993; 122: 1–9.
3 Quinton P. Cystic fibrosis: a disease in electrolyte transport. *FASEB J* 1990; 4: 2709–17.
4 Welsh M. Abnormal regulation of ion channels in cystic fibrosis epithelia. *FASEB J* 1990; 4: 2718–25.
5 Kerem B, Rommens JM, Buchanan JA, et al. Identification of the cystic fibrosis gene: genetic analysis. *Science* 1989; 245: 1073–9.
6 Bear CE, Li C, Kartner N, et al. Purification and functional reconstruction of the cystic fibrosis transmembrane conductance regulator. *Cell* 1992; 66: 809–18.
7 Kopelman H, Durie P, Gaskin K, Weizman Z, Forstner G. Pancreatic fluid and protein hyperconcentration in cystic fibrosis. *N Engl J Med* 1985; 312: 329–34.
8 Durie P, Gaskin K, Kopelman H, Weizman Z, Forstner G. Pancreatic function-testing in cystic fibrosis. *J Pediatr Gastroenterol Nutr* 1984; 3 (suppl 1): S89–98.

9 Gaskin K, Durie P, Lee L, Hill R, Forstner G. Colipase and lipase secretion in childhood onset of pancreatic insufficiency: delineation of patients with steatorrhea with relative colipase deficiency. *Gastroenterology* 1984; **86**: 1–7.

10 Cleghorn GJ, Shepherd RW, Holt TL. The use of a synthetic prostaglandin E1 analogue as an adjunct to pancreatic enzyme replacement in cystic fibrosis. *Scand J Gastroenterol* 1988; **143** (suppl): 142–7.

11 Cox KL, Isenberg JN, Ament ME. Gastric acid hypersecretion in cystic fibrosis. *J Pediatr Gastroenterol Nutr* 1982; **16**: 554–7.

12 Kopelman H, Corey M, Gaskin K, Durie P, Weizman Z, Forstner G. Impaired chloride secretion, as well as bicarbonate secretion, underlies the fluid secretory defect in the cystic fibrosis pancreas. *Gastroenterology* 1988; **95**: 349–55.

13 Gaskin K, Gurwitz D, Durie P, Corey M, Levison H, Forstner G. Improved respiratory prognosis in cystic fibrosis patients with normal fat absorption. *J Pediatr* 1982; **100**: 857–62.

14 Durie P, Kopelman H, Corey M, Laufer D, Forstner G. Pathophysiology of the exocrine pancreas in cystic fibrosis. In: Mastella G, Quinton PM, eds. *Cellular and molecular basis of cystic fibrosis.* San Francisco: San Francisco Press, 1988: 186–90.

15 Taylor CJ, Baxter PS, Hardcastle J, Hardcastle PT. Failure to induce secretion in jejunal biopsies from children with cystic fibrosis. *Gut* 1988; **29**: 957–62.

16 Baxter PS, Wilson AJ, Read NW, Hardcastle J, Hardcastle PT, Taylor CJ. Abnormal jejunal potential difference in cystic fibrosis. *Lancet* 1989; **i**: 464–6.

17 Berschneider HM, Knowles MR, Azizkhan RG, Boucher RC, Tobey NA, Orlando RC, Powell DW. Altered intestinal chloride transport in cystic fibrosis. *FASEB J* 1988; **2**: 2625–9.

18 de Jonge HR, Tilley B, Scholte B, Bijman J, Hoogeveen AT, Sinaasappel M, Veeze H. In: *Proceedings of gastrointestinal epithelium.* Paris: INSERM, 1989: 114–8.

19 Durie P. Gastrointestinal motility disorders in cystic fibrosis. In: Milla PJ, ed. *Disorders of gastrointestinal motility in childhood.* Chichester: John Wiley, 1988: 91–9.

20 Cleghorn GJ, Stringer DA, Forstner G, Durie P. Treatment of the distal intestinal obstruction syndrome in cystic fibrosis with a balanced intestinal lavage solution. *Lancet* 1986; **i**: 8–11.

21 Weizman Z, Durie P, Kopelman H, Vesely S, Forstner G. Bile acid secretion in cystic fibrosis-evidence for a primary defect. *Gut* 1986; **27**: 1362–8.

22 Cohn JA, Strong TV, Picciotto MR, Nairn AC, Collins FS, Fitz JG. Localization of the cystic fibrosis transmembrane conductance regulator in human bile duct epithelial cells. *Gastroenterology* 1993; **106**: 1857–64.

23 Fitz JG, Basavappa S, McGill JM, Melhus O, Cohn JA. Regulation of membrane chloride currents in rat bile duct epithelial cells. *J Clin Invest* 1993; **91**: 319–28.

24 Gaskin KJ, Waters DLM, Howman-Giles R, *et al.* Liver disease and common bile duct stenosis in cystic fibrosis. *N Engl J Med* 1988; **318**: 340–6.

25 Strandvik B, Hjelte L, Gabrielsson N, Glaumann H. Sclerosing cholangitis in cystic fibrosis. *Scand J Gastroenterol Suppl* 1988; **143**: 121–4.

26 Stringer MD, Price JF, Mowat AP, Howard ER. Liver cirrhosis in cystic fibrosis. *Arch Dis Child* 1993; **69**: 407.

27 Colombo C, Setchell KR, Podda M, Crosignani A, Roda A, Curcio L, *et al.* Effects of ursodeoxycholic acid therapy for liver disease associated with cystic fibrosis. *J Pediatr* 1990; **117**: 482–9.

28 Cotting J, Lentze MJ, Reichen J. Effects of ursodeoxycholic acid treatment on nutrition and liver function in patients with cystic fibrosis and longstanding cholestasis. *Gut* 1990; **31**: 918–21.

29 Colombo C, Castellani MR, Balistreri WF, Seregni E, Assaisso ML, Giunta A. Scintigraphic documentation of an improvement in hepatobiliary excretory

function after treatment with ursodeoxycholic acid in patients with cystic fibrosis and associated liver disease. *Hepatology* 1992; **15**: 677–84.

30 Shepherd RW, Holt TL, Vasques-Velasquez L, *et al.* Increased energy expenditure in young children with cystic fibrosis. *Lancet* 1988; **i**: 1300–3.

31 Shepherd R, Cooksley WGE, Cook WDD. Improved growth and clinical nutritional therapy in cystic fibrosis. *J Pediatr* 1980; **97**: 351–6.

32 Mansell AL, Andersen JC, Muttart CR, *et al.* Short-term pulmonary effects of total parenteral nutrition in children with cystic fibrosis. *J Pediatr* 1984; **104**: 700–5.

33 Scott RB, O'Laughlin EV, Gall DG. Gastroesophageal reflux in patients with cystic fibrosis. *J Pediatr* 1985; **106**: 223–7.

34 Levy LD, Durie PR, Pencharz PB, Corey ML. Effects of long-term nutritional rehabilitation on body composition and clinical status in malnourished children and adolescents with cystic fibrosis. *J Pediatr* 1985; **107**: 225–30.

35 Boland MP, Stoski DS, MacDonald NE, Soucy P, Patrick J. Chronic jejunostomy feeding with a non-elemental formula in undernourished patients with cystic fibrosis. *Lancet* 1986; **i**: 232–4.

36 Drury D, Pianosi P, Kopelman H, Charge D, Coates A. The effect of nutritional status on respiratory muscle strength and work capacity in cystic fibrosis. *Pediatr Res* 1990; **27**: 104A.

I thank the Canadian Cystic Fibrosis Foundation for financial support. I currently hold a Chercheur Boursier from the Fonds du Recherche en Santé du Québec.

8 Transplantation

J DARK, P CORRIS

The prevalence of cystic fibrosis is rising, principally because of improvements in survival, and this prevalence is expected to continue to rise over the next 10 years.[1] Pulmonary disease continues to be the leading cause of morbidity and mortality, being responsible for 97% of all deaths and 75% of all hospital admissions.[2] It is no surprise therefore that cystic fibrosis is a major indication for lung transplantation. The registry of the International Society for Heart and Lung Transplantation shows that 38% of all bilateral lung transplants and 16% of all heart and lung transplants have been carried out for cystic fibrosis;[3] in children 61% of all lung transplantations are for cystic fibrosis. Heart lung transplantation or double or bilateral lung transplantation offer new hope for patients with end stage pulmonary disease. In this chapter we review the current status of lung transplantation in cystic fibrosis.

Selection criteria and indications

Patients with cystic fibrosis present a formidable challenge to lung transplantation. The presence of sepsis throughout the respiratory tract, nutritional deficiencies, coexisting gastrointestinal disease and possibly diabetes all militate against successful transplantation, but perhaps because patients are young with extensive experience of hospitals and doctors, and good compliance results in those with cystic fibrosis are as good as those in patients with other indications.[1] Selection of patients is crucial to this success and there are a number of contraindications.

Disability and life expectancy

Transplantation should be considered when there is increasing frequency or duration of hospital admissions, more refractory

120

> ## Patients considered for transplantation
> - Increasing frequency and duration of hospital admissions
> - FEV_1 less than 30% of predicted value
> - $PaCO_2$ of >6.5 kPa

infections, and a progressive decline in weight and lung function despite maximal nutritional support and physiotherapy. Patients with a forced expiratory volume in one second (FEV_1) of less than 30% of the predicted value and a $PaCO_2$ of over 6.5 kPa had a mortality of more than half over a two year period.[4] The FEV_1 proved to be the most significant predictor of mortality, in keeping with similar studies in chronic obstructive pulmonary disease.[5] A fall in FEV_1 to below 30% of the predicted value is usually considered an indication for referral, but in practice it is experience of frequent and poorly controlled infections that tend to precipitate contact with the transplant centre. The onset of hypercarbia and an increasing requirement for oxygen are further indicators of poor prognosis.

A precise estimate of an individual patient's prognosis is difficult to judge despite these general recommendations and there is still room for the experienced physician to make an educated estimate on all the available data, particularly the rate of deterioration. It is important to stress that only patients who seriously want a transplant should be considered for referral and that no patients should be persuaded to have transplants against their wishes.

Systemic disease

The presence of other organ dysfunction in addition to respiratory failure may preclude lung transplantation. Good renal and hepatic function are essential if the patient is to tolerate cyclosporin toxicity. The creatinine clearance or glomerular filtration rate as estimated by the ^{51}Cr-EDTA technique should be more than 50ml/minute. Only minor abnormalities of liver function are acceptable. In particular, impaired coagulation or portal hypertension detected by reverse blood flow in the portal vein on ultrasonography or oesophageal varices in a patient with a large spleen preclude transplantation of the lungs alone. A few patients have undergone heart, lung, and liver transplantation[1] but this may not be justified with the current shortage of donor organs.

Patients with cystic fibrosis commonly have nasal polyps and

121

> ## Contraindications to lung transplantation
>
> - Other systemic disease particularly renal
> - Impaired coagulation
> - Oesophageal varices
> - Enlarged spleen
> - Portal hypertension
> - Aspergilloma
> - Need for mechanical ventilation

bacterial sinusitis together with colonisation with *Pseudomonas aeruginosa*. Antibiotics may be given by aerosol through a full mask to reduce the bacterial load in the upper respiratory tract before transplantation. Symptomatic sinusitis is a surprisingly uncommon problem postoperatively and we have not found it necessary to perform drainage and curettage for asymptomatic sinus disease. Diabetes mellitus, providing it is well controlled and not associated with vascular complications, is not a contraindication.

Cardiac disease

Coronary disease, perhaps because of malabsorption and low lipid concentrations, is virtually unknown in these patients. The presence of cor pulmonale is not a contraindication to successful lung transplantation; the right ventricular performance returns to normal after transplantation of a pulmonary vascular bed with normal resistance.[6] It is important to confirm normal left ventricular function by echocardiography.

Nutritional state

All recipients lose weight during the severely catabolic phase early after transplantation and appreciable preoperative nutritional deficiency increases postoperative risks. Patients with cystic fibrosis who are malnourished must have their nutrition improved. They should have a good calorie intake, optimal enzyme supplementation (which may be improved with the addition of histamine H_2 antagonist) and meticulous control of diabetes. Overnight supplementation either through a nasogastric tube or gastrostomy is particularly effective.

Aspergillus and tuberculosis

The presence of an aspergilloma is a contraindication to lung transplantation. It is difficult to remove the cavity intact and the resultant spillage represents an overwhelming fungal load in an immunosuppressed patient which leads to fungal empyema. Patients with allergic bronchopulmonary aspergillosis or sputum cultures that grow *Aspergillus* may have a successful transplant because the colonising load of *Aspergillus* is so much less. Patients who do have *Aspergillus* in their sputum may benefit from nebulised amphotericin or itraconazole to try and reduce the load. Active mycobacterial infection, including atypical mycobacteria, should be fully treated before the patient can have a transplant.

Burkholderia cepacia

Many patients with end stage disease are colonised by multiply resistant organisms, particularly *B cepacia*. The results of transplantation in this setting are not very good and several centres regard the presence of such organisms as a contraindication.[7] Our policy has been to accept such patients if they lack any other major contraindications and if there is at least one combination of antibiotics to which the organism is partly sensitive.

Previous surgery and pleurodesis

Bleeding from vascular adhesions, which may follow recurrent respiratory infections or may be iatrogenic, can be a major problem particularly when the heart lung transplant is performed through a median sternotomy. A total pleurectomy is probably still a complete contraindication. Lesser degrees of pleurodesis, particularly if the extrapleural plane is intact, can be dealt with by a patient surgeon. The transverse thoracotomy, or "clamshell" incision is particularly useful for this.

Psychological factors

Lung transplantation imposes an enormous stress on patients and their families. Going on the waiting list for a transplant implies that life expectancy is limited and there is a serious risk of death. All involved must understand the risks involved as well as the potential advantages, and the potential recipient must be well motivated. A supportive family or circle of friends is almost essential and underlying psychiatric illness or a background of alcohol or drug abuse are contraindications.

Ventilation

The need for mechanical ventilation is ominous and suggests that the patient will die before the lung can be transplanted. In our view intubated patients who have not been fully assessed should not be accepted for transplantation. Some units will accept patients on mechanical ventilation if they have previously been assessed[8] but the outcome is not as good as for elective patients.[3] Nasal ventilation may be used as a bridge to transplantation in selected patients who develop life-threatening respiratory failure and this mode of support does not seem to affect the outcome adversely.[9]

Discrepancy between donors and recipients

Despite an increase in the number of transplant programmes and a high level of public awareness there is a continuing fall in the number of organs available. The number of isolated lung transplants done in the United Kingdom fell by over 20% between 1994 and 1995. It is clearly necessary to restrict patients going on the waiting list to those who stand a realistic chance both of surviving until a transplant and having a successful outcome afterwards. Despite this there is a considerable attrition rate (Figure 8.1).

Transplant operation and postoperative care

Choice of procedure

The combined heart lung transplant was introduced in 1981 for pulmonary vascular disease, and was applied to a variety of other

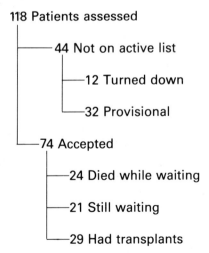

Figure 8.1 Outcome of assessment for cystic fibrosis at Freeman Hospital.

respiratory diseases within a few years.[10] It is a relatively straightforward operation, with a limited number of anastomoses (trachea, aorta, and right atrium) and reliable airway healing. Leaving the heart attached to the pair of lungs kept the donor trachea viable with a blood supply from coronary-bronchial collaterals. It did, however, become apparent that this was the only reason to transplant the heart as the heart that was removed from the recipient (at least in those with cystic fibrosis) was almost invariably normal. The wastage of donor organs was lessened if this heart was given to a cardiac recipient, the so-called "domino procedure," but it remained illogical to transplant the heart only for surgical convenience.

The transplantation of the pair of lungs alone with a tracheal anastomosis — the "enbloc double lung transplant" — was developed by the Toronto group.[11] Unfortunately the heart was usually denervated by the extensive dissection[12] and tracheal healing was not reliable.[13] This latter problem can be solved by surgical revascularisation of the bronchial arteries.[14] It is technically demanding and other potential advantages such as better ciliary function, less infection, and a reduced incidence of obliterative bronchiolitis have yet to be confirmed.

An alternative is to place the bronchial anastomosis closer to the lung parenchyma, either as the "bibronchial" anastomosis favoured by some French groups[15] or as the sequential single or bilateral lung transplant with anastomosis at the hilum for airway, artery, and vein.[16] Coupled with the transverse or "clamshell" incision which gives wonderful access, particularly to the vascular adhesions encountered when removing the lungs, this bilateral lung transplant is our procedure of choice. A number of series have been published with results as good as the best achieved after heart lung transplant.[16–18]

It is clearly necessary to remove both heavily infected lungs but there are occasional patients with such asymmetrically sized pleural cavities, perhaps as a result of previous lobectomy or prolonged collapse, that implantation of a pair of lungs is impossible. The options include transplantation of just one lobe, or a pneumonectomy followed by contralateral single lung transplant, an approach we have successfully applied in one case.[19]

Donor selection and size matching

Our current donor criteria are given in the box. Good gas exchange in the donor is the most important determinant of early

---

Donor criteria

- ABO compatibility
- Age < 65 years
- CMV match to recipient
- Size match on height (within 10%)
- PaO$_2$ < 40 kPa on FI02 < 1.0
- Clear chest radiograph
- Low airway pressure on ventilator
- No history of chest surgery or injury
- Non-purulent tracheal aspirate

---

postoperative performance of the transplanted lungs.[20] We try to match (within 20%) the presumed total lung capacity of the donor (as predicted from height and weight), to the predicted total lung capacity of the recipient. The actual total lung capacity is usually greater, allowing some leeway for slightly larger lungs. After pretreatment with steroids and prostacyclin or one of its analogues the lungs are flushed with a cold solution and transported, still inflated, to the recipient hospital. Ischaemic times of up to eight hours are tolerated with this technique.[21] Donor and recipient must be ABO blood group compatible and we attempt to match for cytomegalovirus (CMV) status.

Anaesthesia and surgery — bilateral lung transplant

In the original descriptions[16] great emphasis was placed on avoidance of cardiopulmonary bypass, so a double lumen endotracheal tube to allow ventilation of one lung together with the means to monitor cardiac performance such as a Swan Ganz catheter and transoesophageal echocardiography, were thought essential. One lung, usually the right, was removed and replaced, followed by the same on the left. The pulmonary venous anastomoses on the left are particularly difficult in this setting, entailing much retraction on the heart despite considerable lateral extension of the transverse incision. These difficulties have led us to evolve a technique with extensive reliance on cardiopulmonary bypass, allowing a single lumen endotracheal tube, and dispensing with extensive monitoring.[21]

The chest is opened through a transverse incision in the fifth interspace, with transsection of the sternum. Pleural adhesions are taken down before heparinisation and the lungs are then removed at each hilum. The heart is allowed to beat on bypass but does no work. There is excellent access for anastomoses at bronchus, left atrium, and pulmonary artery. The new lungs are kept immersed in cold saline until implantation on both sides is complete. They are then reperfused simultaneously in a controlled fashion, and then the heart easily takes over the circulation. Though there are theoretical disadvantages of bypass in lung transplantation,[22] early function is usually excellent. The potential problem of bleeding with systemic heparinisation has been much diminished with the use of antifibrinolytic agent aprotinin[23] and re-exploration for bleeding has been required in only one of 40 patients in our series of bilateral lung transplants. This contrasts with a re-exploration rate of up to 30% after heart and lung transplantation.[24]

Early postoperative care

Postoperative pain is a particular disadvantage of the clamshell incision, and epidural analgesia is useful. If gas exchange is good and the patient is haemodynamically stable, weaning from the ventilator can start within a few hours. Transfer from the intensive care unit is usually achieved within 48–72 hours by which time all drains have been removed. Oral intake can start at about the same time and feeding through a gastrotomy, if in place, can usefully be restarted. Pancreatic enzyme supplementation together with histamine H_2 antagonists are added from the start. Meconium ileus equivalent can be a problem and prophylaxis with n-acetylcysteine, or more usually a properistaltic agent such as cisapride is routine. Perioperative stress together with high doses of corticosteroids often uncover glucose intolerance even if the patient was not previously diabetic and this requires standard management with an infusion of short-acting insulin.

Detection and treatment of postoperative infections

The organisms and their sensitivities harboured by the recipients, are identified at the time of assessment and this information should be kept up to date by the referring hospital. Sputum is recultured on admission for transplant and bronchoalveolar lavage of the recipient lungs is always done after they are removed. In over half the cases a strain of *Pseudomonas* is found in the lavage fluid which is not present in the simple sputum culture. Similarly at least

30% of donor lungs will be contaminated by both bacteria and fungi. This should be identified by lavage of the donor lungs and antibiotic treatment altered accordingly. An antifungal agent should be added if there are any fungi in the lavage fluid because of the risk of colonisation and subsequent disruption of vascular suture lines.

Our standard prophylactic antibiotics for these patients are flucloxacillin, metronidazole, and aztreonam but they may be varied in the light of previous information or after the operation when the most recent results from the donor and the recipient are available. Antipseudomonal antibiotics are continued for at least seven days, supplemented by nebulised colistin except in patients with organisms, particularly *B cepacia*, which have previously been shown to be resistant to colistin.

A further bronchoalveolar lavage is done at the time of the routine seven day biopsy and in response to any unexplained pyrexia or reduction in pulmonary function. Subsequent antibiotics can therefore be chosen carefully but the mere presence of *Pseudomonas* in an otherwise well patient is not an indication for treatment.

Viral infections

Most patients with cystic fibrosis have never been exposed to CMV and ideally all such serologically negative recipients should receive organs from CMV negative donors. If transfused blood is screened for CMV, postoperative infection with that virus is rare.

If lungs from a CMV positive donor are transplanted there is a risk of donor transmitted disease. Our policy is to give prophylactic immunoglobulin which, although expensive (about £3000 for a seven week course at 1995 prices), is effective.[25] There is usually a primary infection which manifests itself 40–50 days after transplantation with a fever accompanied by excretion of CMV into lavage fluid or urine and seroconversion with the appearance of IgM. There may be infiltrates in the chest radiograph and the characteristic histological appearance ("owls eye" bodies) in the transbronchial biopsy specimen, but this is often a self-limiting illness. Treatment with the specific anti-CMV agent ganciclovir is required for symptomatic pneumonitis or other serious organ involvement. Prophylactic ganciclovir has been recommended in this group of patients[26] but is no more effective than immunoglobulin and may predispose to recurrent infections.

Such patients are also at risk from infection from herpes viruses and we continue prophylactic acyclovir in a dose of 200 mg three times daily for three months. This treatment may also offer some protection against Epstein-Barr virus lymphoproliferative disorders.

Immunosuppression

Most centres use a classic three drug regimen consisting of Cyclosporin, Azathioprine, and corticosteroids. Because early renal function is important in the first few days after transplantation, early cyclosporin doses are low and initial protection is achieved with antithymocyte globulin. Flow cytometry should be used to monitor the absolute T cell count (as indicated by the CD3 marker), keeping this less than 50 000 cells mm^{-3}. This drug is used for three days and continued only if adequate concentrations of cyclosporin cannot be attained. Longer courses of antithymocyte globulin have no proven advantage and may predispose the patient to subsequent lymphoproliferative disease. The standard immunosuppression regimen is shown in Table 8.1. Corticosteroids are used both perioperatively and in relatively high doses during the first few weeks. This routine has not been associated with impaired bronchial healing.[27]

Long term management of patients with cystic fibrosis after transplantation

Surveillance for pulmonary rejection and infection

Patients are monitored clinically, radiographically, and by pulmonary function testing. Episodes of infection and acute

Table 8.1   Lung transplantation for cystic fibrosis

	Immunosuppression regimen	
● Cyclosporin	–	Preoperative oral dose of 4 mg/kg
	–	Postoperative intravenous infusion for five days
	–	Trough level 400 mg/l for six months (Neoral since May 1995)
● Azathioprine	–	Preoperative oral dose of 4 mg/kg
	–	Postoperatively 0–2 mg/kg
	–	White cell count 4–6 × $10^9$1
● Corticosteroids	–	10 mg/kg Before reperfusion
	–	2 mg/kg Eight hourly in first 24 hours
	–	1 mg/kg Tailed off over 14 days
	–	0.2 mg/kg For six months

rejection may present with identical changes and should be investigated by bronchoscopy with bronchoalveolar lavage and transbronchial lung biopsy. The principal cause of early post-operative death is infection and bacterial pneumonia is reported to affect up to 35% of patients in the first three months.[28] Patients with cystic fibrosis do not have a higher incidence of bacterial pneumonia than recipients with other conditions although the incidence of pseudomonal infections is higher. There is debate about the value of surveillance biopsies carried out in patients who are clinically well. A recent study showed that 20% of patients have clinically covert rejection of Grade 2 or greater up to six months after transplantation. Further studies from our group have shown that acute rejection that persists beyond the first month, and episodes of organising pneumonia are risk factors for the subsequent development of chronic graft dysfunction as a result of obliterative bronchiolitis.[29] Surveillance biopsies may help stratify the intensity of immunosuppression that is required to prevent obliterative bronchiolitis, but positive evidence to support this is currently lacking.

Chronic complications after transplantation

Obliterative bronchiolitis

This process may be defined functionally by the development of progressive irreversible airflow obstruction that does not respond to corticosteroids. Histological examination shows obliteration of bronchioles by organising fibrosis associated with fibroblasts and mononuclear cells. The small bronchioles are left as fibrous bands extending out of the pleura with associated dilatation and bronchiectasis more proximally. Obliterative bronchiolitis is the most important long term complication that limits survival after transplantation, affecting 30%–50% of patients after five years.[30] When established, the condition is progressive and although intensification of immunosuppression may reduce the functional decline, only occasionally is it reversed. Much research in lung transplantation is directed towards preventing this complication and how to identify patients at risk at an early stage. Management of an established case includes postural drainage to increase clearance of secretions, nebulised antibiotics including colistin and tobramycin to try and reduce the colonising load of *Pseudomonas*, which is commonly associated with bronchiectasis, and bronchiolitis. The onset of obliterative bronchiolitis has a major psychological impact on patients, who require compassion and tender handling.

The only established treatment for obliterative bronchiolitis is retransplantation. The results are not good[31] and this should be applied only to carefully selected patients, if at all. Because of bronchiectasis and recolonisation with *Pseudomonas* it is usually necessary to remove all the pulmonary tissue and at least to do a second bilateral lung transplant.

Post–transplant lymphoproliferative disease

Immunosuppression and the Ebstein–Barr virus (EBV) have been linked to the development of lymphoproliferative disease. The control of EBV infection is mediated primarily by EBV specific cytotoxic T-lymphocytes and by specific antibodies directed towards the viral antigens. In immunosuppressed patients the balance between viral proliferation and T-cell control is shifted. EBV replicates in oropharyngeal epithelial cells and infects B-lymphocytes. The infested cells may lyse with subsequent release of mature viral particles, or survive and have viral DNA incorporated into the host genome.[32] A range of lymphoproliferative disorders from benign polyclonal B cell hyperplasia to the classic monoclonal malignant lymphoma may occur.[33] Treatment is with high doses of acyclovir and a reduction in immunosuppression, and the results are usually favourable. Patients with more malignant disease, usually the monoclonal form, may require chemotherapy and the results are often disappointing. Endobronchial disease is sometimes seen after lung transplantation and is perhaps caused by the latent EBV genome in lymphoid tissue associated with the graft bronchus. Post-transplant lymphoproliferative disease in a lung transplant recipient almost invariably presents first in the transplanted organ.

Osteoporosis

There is increasing evidence of osteoporosis and osteoporotic vertebral collapse in patients after transplantation. Patients with cystic fibrosis are particularly at risk as most will have established osteoporosis before transplantation.[34] The routine use of oral corticosteroids and the need for the frequent courses of high doses of pulsed methylprednisolone given intravenously increases the risk. The optimum management of such patients is under investigation and most units use biphosphonates and calcium supplementation at present.

Results

Regardless of the procedure used, experienced centres report a 70%–75% one year survival after transplantation for patients with cystic fibrosis. There is an inexorable attrition rate related primarily to obliterative bronchiolitis, resulting in a five year survival of 40%–50%.[26] The quality of life of survivors is usually excellent with a return to normal respiratory function. Most of the patients are young and are able to take part in a full range of leisure and professional activities. A number of successful pregnancies have occurred in this group. Despite the fact that survival is limited for most of them transplant is nearly always regarded as a rewarding experience.

References

1 Geddes DM, Hodson ME. Cystic fibrosis: future trends in care. *Thorax* 1988; **43**: 869–71.
2 Penketh ARC, Wise A, Mearns MB, Hodson ME, Balten JC. Cystic fibrosis in adolescents and adults. *Thorax* 1987; **42**: 526–32.
3 Hosenpud JD, Novick RJ, Breen T, Daily OP. The registry of the International Society of Heart and Lung Transplantation. Eleventh official report 1994. *J Heart & Lung Transplant* 1994; **13**: 561–70.
4 Kerem E, Reisman J, Cory M, Canny GJ, Levison H. Prediction of mortality in patients with cystic fibrosis. *N Engl J Med* 1992; **326**: 1187.
5 Anthonisen NR, Wright EC, Hodgkin JE, *et al*. Prognosis in chronic obstructive pulmonary disease. *Am Rev Respir Dis* 1986; **133**: 14–20.
6 Doig JC, Corris PA, Hilton CJ, Dark JH, Bexton RS. The effect of single lung transplantation on pulmonary hypertension in patients with end-stage fibrosing lung disease. *Br Heart J* 1991; **66**: 431–4.
7 Shennib H, Adoumie R, Noirclerc M. Current status of lung transplantation for cystic fibrosis. *Arch Intern Med* 1992; **152**: 1585–8.
8 Massard G, Shennib H, Metras D, Chamboulives J, Viard L, Mulder DS, Tcherverkov CI, Morin J-F, Givdicelli R, Noirclerc M. Double lung transplantation in mechanically ventilated cystic fibrosis patients. *Ann Thorac Surg* **55(5)**: 1087–91.
9 Hodson ME, Madden BP, Steven MH, Tsang VT, Yacoub MH. Non invasive mechanical ventilation for cystic fibrosis patients: bridge to transplantation. *Eur Respir J* 1993; **6**: 965–70.
10 Penketh A, Higgenbotham TW, Hakim M, Wallwork J. Heart and lung transplantation in patients with end stage lung disease. *BMJ* 1987; **295**: 311–6.
11 Dark JH, Patterson GA, Al-Jihaihawi AN, Hsu H, Egan T, Cooper JD. Experimental en-block double lung transplantation in dogs. *Ann Thorac Surg* 1996; **42**: 395–8.
12 Schafers HJ, Waxman MB, Patterson GA, Frost AE, Maurer J, Cooper JD, and the Toronto Lung Transplant Group. Cardiac innervation after double lung transplant. *J Thorac Cardiovasc Surg* 1990; **99**: 22–6.
13 Patterson GA, Todd TR, Cooper JD, Pearson FG, Winton TL, Maurer J, and the Toronto Lung Transplant Group. Airway complication after double lung transplantation. *J Thorac Cardiovasc Surg* 1990; **99**: 14–21.
14 Daly RC, McGregor CGA. Routine immediate direct bronchial revascularisation for single lung transplantation. *Ann Thorac Surgery* 1995; **57**: 1446–52.

15 Noirclerc MJ, Metras D, Vaillant A, Dumon JF, Zimmermann JM, Caemano A, Orsoni PC. Bilateral bronchial anastomosis in double lung and heart lung transplantation. *Eur J Cardiothorac Surg* 1990; 4: 314–7.

16 Pasque MK, Cooper JD, Kaiser LR, *et al*. Improved technique for bilateral lung transplantation: rationale and initial clinical experience. *Ann Thorac Surg* 1990; 49: 785–91.

17 Dromer C, Velly JF, Jougon J, Martigne C, Baudet EM, Couraud L. Long term functional results after bilateral lung transplantation. *Ann Thorac Surg* 1993; 56: 68–72.

18 Egan TM, Detterbeck FC, Mill MR, Paradowski LJ, Lackner RP, Ogden WD, Yankaskas JR, Westerman JH, Thompson JT, Weiner MA, Cairns EL, Wilcox BR. Improved results of lung transplantation for patients with cystic fibrosis. *J Thorac Cardiovasc Surg* 1995; 109: 224–35.

19 Forty J, Hasan A, Gould FK, Corris PA, Dark JH. Single lung transplantation with simultaneous contralateral pneumonectomy for cystic fibrosis. *J Heart Lung Transplant* 1994; 13: 727–36.

20 Waller DA, Forty J, Corris PA, Gould FK, Hilton CJ, Dark JH. Determinants of early outcome after lung transplantation. *J Heart Lung Transplant* 1995; 14(suppl): S94.

21 Hasan A, Corris PA, Healy M, *et al*. Bilateral sequential lung transplantation for end-stage septic lung disease. *Thorax* 1995; 50: 565–6.

22 Fullerton DA, McIntyre RC, Mitchell MB, Campbell DN, Grover FL. Lung transplantation with cardiopulmonary bypass exaggerates pulmonary vasomotor dysfunction in the transplanted lung. *J Thorac Cardiovasc Surg* 1995; 109: 212–7.

23 Royston D. High dose aprotinin therapy: a review of the first five years experience. *Journal of Cardiovascular Anaesthesia* 1992; 76–100.

24 Jones K, Higgenbotham T, Wallwork J. Successful heart-lung transplantation for cystic fibrosis. *Chest* 1988; 93: 644–5.

25 Gould FK, Freeman R, Taylor CE, Ashcroft T, Dark JH, Corris PA. Prophylaxis and management of cytomegalovirus after lung transplantation: a review of experience in one centre. *J Heart Lung Transplant* 1993; 12: 695–9.

26 Blumberg EA, Fitzpatrick JM, Stutman PC, Gash S, Brozena SC. CMV prophylaxis does not prevent CMV disease in heart-lung transplant patients. *J Heart Lung Transplant* 1994; 14(suppl): S65.

27 Colquhoun IW, Gascoigne AD, Au J, Corris PA, Hilton CJ, Dark JH. Airway complications following pulmonary transplantation. *Ann Thorac Surg* 1994; 57: 141–5.

28 Dauber JH, Paradis IC, Drummer JS. Infectious complications in pulmonary allograft recipients. *Clin Chest Med* 1990; 11: 291.

29 Milne DS, Gascoigne AD, Ashcroft T, Sviland L, Malcolm A, Corris PA. Organising pneumonia following pulmonary transplantation and the development of obliterative bronchiolitis. *Transplantation* 1994; 57: 1757–62.

30 Madden BP, Hodson ME, Tsang V, Radley-Smith R, Patterson GA, Kaye MP, Menkis AM, McKenzie FN. Intermediate term results of heart-lung transplantation for cystic fibrosis. *Lancet* 1992; 339: 1583–7.

31 Novick RJ, Andressian B, Schafers JH, *et al*. Pulmonary retransplantation for obliterative bronchiolitis. Intermediate-term results of a Northern American-European series. *Journal Thorac Cardiovasc Surg* 1994; 107: 755–63.

32 Hanto DW, Frizzera G, Gajl-Peczalska KJ, *et al*. Epstein-Barr virus, immunodeficiency and B-cell lymphoproliferation. *Transplantation* 1985; 39: 461–72.

33 Nagington J, Gray J. Cyclosporin A. Immunosuppression, Epstein Barr antibody and lymphoma. *Lancet* 1980; i: 536–7.

34 Bachrach L, Loutit C, Moss R, Marcus R. Ostopenia in adults with cystic fibrosis. *Am J Med* 1994; 96: 21–4.

9 Social and psychological perspectives

S WYNN–KNIGHT

In this chapter I will consider the impact of cystic fibrosis on patients and their families. Having a child with cystic fibrosis means learning to live with the uncertainty of chronic disease; the unpredictability of prognosis, and adapting to maintain a life that is as normal as possible. Armour states that "uncertainty is both a curse and a blessing but it has taught us some skills in balancing on a tightrope between hope and despair."[1] In order to live on this tightrope these families need support at a social, psychological, emotional, and clinical level.[2]

It is important for all members of the multidisciplinary cystic fibrosis team to recognise that the components of support are closely related and equally important. Each member has a defined responsibility for an aspect of care, but the clinical nurse specialist can ideally liaise between members of the team and the patients. The nurse specialist must have a detailed knowledge and understanding of all the patients, the families, and the state of their disease. At least one member of the team can therefore consider each patient as a whole, intervening appropriately to ensure high quality care is delivered and anxiety is reduced.

Parents

Consideration for the parents is important as the health of the child profoundly influences the wellbeing of the whole family. Parents who choose to deny the diagnosis or who are unable to express their feelings about their child and the burden of care may

Potential crisis times for parents

- Diagnosis and realisation of the meaning of cystic fibrosis
- Further pregnancies
- Learning to cope with new demands, which may occur each time a new treatment is instigated
- First course of intravenous antibiotics and isolation of new bacteria from the sputum
- Problems with school and employment
- Increasing need for antibiotics
- Change from paediatric to adult care
- Loss of responsibility such as allowing the child to perform their own treatment
- Decisions about transplantation
- Deteriorating health of a sibling with cystic fibrosis, friend, or one's own child
- Death of a sibling with cystic fibrosis, friend, or own child
- Bereavement

be unable to make satisfactory adaptations. Both parents need support and if they are able to adapt their partnership may survive though if only one parent adapts there is often considerable conflict.[3 4] Life with a child with cystic fibrosis is a series of events, each resulting in feelings of loss (Box). The normal reactions include anger, guilt, fear, despair, denial, and sadness,[5] and families may "need permission" to recognise that they are worthy of grief and accept support through such grieving.[6] Grieving helps families to adapt more easily as each loss occurs, leading finally to a state of acceptance. Future losses in families that have been able to adapt are coped with better and the families are able to work more closely with health professionals to provide the best care for their child or children. By contrast suppression of emotions can have physical and psychological effects that lead to unresolved grief,[7] and in such families resentment will often lead to anger which is aimed at the people most involved with caring for their child.

Nurse specialists are "safe" people to be angry with because the family know that they are unlikely to leave. People may be afraid of their own feelings and emotions and need support from a person with whom they feel safe to work through these emotions. It is essential to recognise that such anger is not usually personal and is probably necessary for the family to work through their anger and grieve fully for their losses.

Examples of loss for parents of a child with cystic fibrosis

Diagnosis

Parents often feel the loss of a healthy baby or child at the time of diagnosis.[8] This is accompanied by the realisation that the child has a shortened life expectancy, as well as the guilt of knowing that they passed the cystic fibrosis gene to the child.

Response

Parents may need genetic counselling to understand the recessive mode of inheritance, particularly if they are considering further pregnancies. They may choose prenatal diagnosis and termination if a further baby is found to have cystic fibrosis; this may pose the dilemma of whether a termination devalues the life of the child already born with cystic fibrosis.[3 9] Families also benefit from broader counselling, support, education, and sharing their knowledge and feelings with other affected families.[7]

Difficulties with treatment

For many parents the first treatment hurdle is getting used to giving enzyme supplements. The correct dose may take time to establish, leading to anxiety over the child's eating habits and ability to put on weight. Parents may try hard to encourage the child to eat and feel despair and disbelief when professionals note the failure of the child to grow; this only compounds their feelings of guilt and fear. Such an approach may seem critical and make the situation worse, and children may learn that they have control over their parents because of concerns over poor eating habits. The attitude to physiotherapy may be similar because the parents understand the importance of the treatment but it is difficult to force children to undertake a treatment that they dislike. Parents may experience feelings of guilt when the child is ill, particularly if this leads to admission to hospital and they may also fear that each hospital admission is an indicator of an untimely death.

Response

Members of the cystic fibrosis team should work closely with the parents to overcome the problems. The social worker and the cystic fibrosis nurse specialist, or possibly a psychologist, can offer support to parents by talking through the difficulties. They may be able to break the cycle of parental anxiety and unreasonable control over the parents by the child by admitting the child to hospital or by giving advice to the parents. Physiotherapists can offer the same practical advice and support over difficulties with physiotherapy.

Leading a normal life

A major concern is how a child's needs and treatment can be incorporated into a relatively normal lifestyle. Parents should consider their own needs and those of the siblings of the affected child. The temptation with a chronically sick child is to be over protective, which often leads to resentment and jealousy both from the sibling and the affected child who may wish to be like the unaffected sibling.

Response

Parents should be encouraged to treat children with cystic fibrosis as if they did not have the disease by encouraging participation in activities that are normal for a child without cystic fibrosis of the same age. They should be encouraged to set achievable goals which give them hope for the future and increase the self esteem of both children and parents.

Infection and lung disease

A patient with cystic fibrosis cannot be protected from every infection, though contact with some infections that are recognised to be more serious in cystic fibrosis can sensibly be avoided. (See Chapter 6.)

Response

The nurse specialist, physiotherapist, and other members of the cystic fibrosis team should provide information and advice to parents, general practitioners, teachers, and others involved in the child's care, as a better understanding can improve the care and reduce parental anxiety.[2] Parents need to know when it is necessary to obtain antibiotics and how to get them. Cross infection in the community and in the hospital causes a lot of fear and anxiety and it should be clearly explained to parents exactly what the risk is.

Loss of normal life events

The father of a boy with cystic fibrosis may be deeply affected by the likelihood that his son will be sterile.

The loss of normal life expectancy, both in terms of length,

137

interrupted education, family life, holidays, and career expectations, as well as those of long term relationships and marriage, are losses which affect the parents initially and later have an impact on the patients themselves.[9] These losses are brought back to the parents repeatedly with the realisation that the child will probably die before them, that normal everyday life is likely to be interrupted by medication, the need for physiotherapy and sometimes acute deterioration in health and repeated hospital admissions.

Response

Members of the cystic fibrosis team should listen to the parents to find out what their fears and anxieties are. Parents may well need simple explanations as they may not have understood all the implications of the disease. The professionals must be aware of the messages that the family are getting and ensure that they have a clear and accurate understanding of what is happening to their child at any one time. Repeated explanations may be needed to ensure full understanding. As the disease progresses more complicated explanations may be needed so that the family understand the importance of a particular event — for example, chronic colonisation with *Pseudomonas aeruginosa*, and its implications for the child's health.

Patterson discusses the impact of the relationship between family functioning and the health of the child with cystic fibrosis stating that "Parental coping by getting involved in activities that enhance self esteem, help manage psychological tension, and promote social support appear to benefit the child's health."[10]

This may have a long term impact on the health of the child and its survival. By attention to such detail and the use of graded information the cystic fibrosis team can work with parents to keep them fully informed and to help them make informed decisions about the care of their child. In addition to professionals supporting the family it is important to bear in mind that many parents find discussion of issues that they think peculiar to cystic fibrosis are better dealt with by talking to the parents of another child with cystic fibrosis.

Siblings and the impact of chronic illness

A sibling's response to growing up with chronic illness is unique and individual and depends on multiple variables. Such factors as age, sex, developmental level, and birth order may influence an individual's response to the situation.[11]

The family dynamics, attitudes, and beliefs will also have an impact on the child's response.[12] Whyte discusses the effects of family stress on the healthy sibling particularly when this child becomes the focus of parental distress and anger, often during exacerbations of the child's illness.[3] This stress may place extra responsibility on the well child who is not ready emotionally or developmentally to take on these demands. Rosenstein observed that healthy siblings were angry and resentful of the lack of parental attention they received and were shown to have more difficulties at school.[13] These experiences are likely to create feelings of loss and grief as siblings attempt to grapple with their own emotional feelings about the child with cystic fibrosis, the reduction in parental attention, and disruption to their daily routine. Siblings may be concerned that they will catch the disease or may even wish they had it so that they received more parental attention.

The financial constraints that occur in families with chronically sick children could well affect the healthy siblings.

Case 1

A man of 28 years had just lost his second sibling as a result of cystic fibrosis, both of whom were younger than him. During discussion he stated that he felt guilty because he was well, healthy, and alive; guilty that he did not have cystic fibrosis; and guilty that when he was younger he often got angry with his siblings and sometimes said that he wished they were dead so that he could have some parental attention.

It is the combination of conflicting emotions of jealousy, hatred, anger, fear, and love that caused this young man to distance himself from his family as he grew up, adding further feelings of guilt and neglect to his grief.

Response

It is crucial to involve siblings in the care of the child with cystic fibrosis so that they feel needed and have a sense of belonging. Siblings need explanations given in a way they can understand in order to alleviate their anxieties about themselves and the child with cystic fibrosis. They may benefit from being able to talk about their feelings to someone outside the family, such as the cystic fibrosis nurse, specialist, or social worker.

Lobato states that: "Beginning honest conversation about a difficult topic at an early age will not make a problem disappear but will provide the child with the clear message that problems can be discussed and shared within the family."[14]

If siblings are not able to express their feelings and understand the situation they may become more disruptive and difficult in order to gain attention. This is likely to increase the levels of stress within the family even more. They may even blame themselves for their sibling's illness or death. Lobato discusses the use of sibling workshops as a way of helping them to adjust to life with a chronically sick brother or sister.

Where the family are able to focus their energies on maintaining a positive attitude and a family lifestyle which is as "normal" as possible,[1] rather than focusing on the child's disease and treatment needs, they will be more able to adjust to the situation and meet the needs of all family members.

Finding the balance between the treatment needs of the child with cystic fibrosis and maintaining normality can be very difficult.

This is where support and advice from health care professionals may be invaluable in helping them achieve this balance.

Children with cystic fibrosis

Acceptance of treatment

The child's problems usually begin with learning to accept treatment. This may mean that parents have to find innovative ways of making treatment acceptable rather than a constant battle. Children who learn from an early age to accept physiotherapy and medication as a routine often have less problems than those who

---

Requirements of siblings during their childhoods[14]

- Information on the child's condition, including how it is evaluated and treated
- Open communication within the family about the problem and family members' positive and negative experiences with it
- Recognition by parents of the siblings' own strengths and accomplishments
- Need for "quality time" with their parents on an individual basis
- Contact and support from other siblings and families
- Ways to cope with stressful events such as peer and public reaction, unexpected disruptions to family plans, and extra home responsibility.

---

receive irregular treatment. There may be difficulties when children start school, because treatment has to be incorporated into the school day. There may be difficulty with taking essential medication at school, and because children realise that they are different from their peers they may be reluctant to accept medication and physiotherapy. Some children are teased at school because they need to take medication, have smelly stools, or because of their chronic cough. Misinformed teachers may also make school difficult for children with cystic fibrosis by making them feel different or by seeming to be critical of illness or absence. These pressures may cause children to avoid treatment or refuse to go to school, making the problem worse (Box).

Many of these problems can be alleviated by providing teachers and other children with information about cystic fibrosis; this encourages them to help to support children with cystic fibrosis, and to treat them as normal people. Children with cystic fibrosis should be encouraged to discuss fears and anxieties so that they can learn more effective methods of dealing with the implications of their disorder. This should include encouragement to be involved in their own care as early as possible so that they learn to take responsibility for their treatment. When additional treatment is necessary and hospital admissions become a feature of care it is important to explain to these children why they have the treatment and what it involves.

Play therapy is an important part of encouraging children to express their fears and anxieties about their treatment. "For many children and most children at certain times some features of their environment presses too hardly upon them, and the way out that is left to them is the recreation in play of the same environment, but with the painful features remodelled to their heart's desire."[15]

Helping a child to cope with losses involves listening and finding out the nature of their anxieties as well as working through potential solutions.[16] Problems may be emotional, and children may need someone from outside the family with whom to discuss fears and anxieties to enable them to develop effective coping methods to face future losses.[9]

Case 1

A three year old boy was admitted to hospital because he refused to take pancreatic enzymes. The nurse specialist spent time explaining why enzymes are important. For two days he took no enzymes and gradually developed severe abdominal pain associated with offensive smelling stools. He was given the option of stomach ache or taking the enzymes. He agreed with some reluctance and needed a lot of encouragement. The stomach pain resolved, but after a further day of refusing enzymes it returned and he recognised the association between enzymes and freedom from discomfort. He then started regular treatment with enzymes having learned the clear implications of not taking them.

Adolescence and cystic fibrosis

Adolescence is a period of physical, mental, and social change.[10] To the individual child it is a time of self discovery and erratic, extreme, and often rebellious behaviour which is a way of adapting to such changes. For adolescents with chronic illness there are extra problems to cope with.

The losses experienced during adolescence largely relate to poor self esteem secondary to poor growth, weight gain, cough and production of sputum, and the constant need for medication.[8] The further problem of delayed sexual development is often a feature, particularly in boys. Anxiety can be caused by separation from peers at school or family during periods in hospital and the disease may be perceived as some form of punishment. The struggle for independence — a normal part of adolescence — may be considerably more difficult to achieve for children who have been dependent on their parents for many years. It may be made worse by parallel parental anxiety about the ability of adolescents to care adequately for their own health. Adolescents need an opportunity

---

Losses that may be experienced during childhood

- Realisation that child is different from peers because of treatments and need for medication
- Disruption of education by absence from school through illness and hospital attendance
- Reduced expectations because of limitations of the disease
- Loss of self esteem because of teasing about coughing, sputum production, poor growth, and being different
- Loss of control because of the need to adhere to treatment
- Loss of feeling of normality because the child is treated differently from other siblings and peers
- Loss caused by separation from parents when the child is admitted to hospital and the parents cannot be there
- Loss of friendships either through death or parental separation from peers with cystic fibrosis

---

to experience control and autonomy which may ease their feelings of uncertainty and turmoil.[17]

Response

There is a need for open discussion with patients about the impact of their disease. They will need help to gain independence — for example, learning self-physiotherapy and taking responsibility for their own medication. An opportunity to talk with other patients with cystic fibrosis is often helpful in coping with the difficulties, and may reduce feelings of isolation, difference, and loss. Parents who try to protect their children from issues such as life expectancy, death, and male sterility, may cause later problems when the patient finds out the reality of these problems; they may be angry at not having been made aware of them at an earlier age. With professional and lay support, as in other age groups, adolescents can learn to adapt and improve the quality of their existence, but some will refuse to accept help and compliance with treatment may be poor leading to rapid deterioration in health. The relationship between the ability to comply with treatment and an individual's psychological state is discussed by Nichols.[18]

Case 2

A rebellious 14 year old girl "knew about cystic fibrosis" and considered that physiotherapy and antibiotics were a waste of time. She did not take her medication, and despite producing large quantities of tenacious purulent sputum, refused physiotherapy or admission to hospital for intravenous treatment with antibiotics. When she was admitted with haemoptysis all the members of the clinical team attempted to discuss the importance of compliance with treatment. The nurse specialist explained the process and the potential consequences of no treatment. The greatest impact came from discussion with another patient who was terminally ill and who confided in the girl that she believed that she was dying because she had not complied with treatment. The girl left hospital intending to start physiotherapy. After her second admission to hospital she started to take her own care seriously, doing physiotherapy two to three times a day and taking her medication including overnight nasogastric tube feeding. She continued to comply with her treatment until she died two and a half years later.

Denial had been a coping mechanism in the girl's family. Her parents had denied the need for treatment during her childhood and that attitude had passed on to her. The earlier availability of support at the time of diagnosis may well have helped the family to adapt to a more healthy and positive approach to their daughter's disease which might have affected the girl's length and quality of life.

Response

Teenagers require an approach that is aimed at improving their self esteem and which gives them hope and reasons to carry out their treatment. They need to build relationships with the team based on honesty and trust which encourage them to make informed decisions about treatment. Additional support should prepare them for taking on the responsibility of their treatment with a view to living independently from their parents, if this is appropriate. It is also important to encourage a positive attitude towards planning for the future with regards to education, career, and relationships. Although some patients will not achieve their goals they should be encouraged to live as normal a life as possible. A positive approach does not mean that the difficult aspects of the disease are ignored, but comes from personal growth and understanding of the disease derived from different experiences of loss.

Transfer from adolescence to adulthood

Transferring from paediatric to adult care may be difficult for both patients and their families. The thought of care from a new team of professionals may be daunting, particularly if this means moving to a new hospital. The transition period can be eased by combined paediatric and adult clinics which give patients an opportunity to get to know the team who treat the adults.[19-21] Adolescents may also need help to release the parental attachment so that they are able to follow their chosen career, particularly where this means moving away from home. In encouraging independence, the adult team can play a major part in inspiring individual patients to take responsibility for their care. This requires professionals with a positive attitude and a good understanding of the needs of young adults. Conveying detailed information will help to improve the self confidence of the patients and this will often be supplemented by gaining self confidence from meeting other adults with cystic fibrosis.

Adults with cystic fibrosis

Adults with cystic fibrosis have many difficulties, particularly in terms of choices to be made about their lives. A major decision is whether or not to live independently of parents. The choice of career may be affected because of the limitations imposed by the disease or the lack of available employment. Some choose between career, social life and the needs of treatment, while others learn to balance time and energy among all three. Some adults deny the presence of disease and may consider the best quality of life for them is a shorter life expectancy with little or no treatment compared with longer life expectancy and the compromise between the needs of treatment, career and social life. "Quality of life is as important as prolongation of life."[22]

Some patients choose their friends from among peers with cystic fibrosis because they gain support, friendship, and a greater understanding from others with the same problem, while others will opt for minimal contact with other patients with cystic fibrosis. Finding a partner may bring specific problems and the question of when to tell the prospective partner that you have cystic fibrosis and how much to tell often arises. In this area the health professional should be sensitive to the needs of each individual patient. Some patients avoid getting involved in relationships because of poor self esteem or fear of rejection. Part of this may be that they are reluctant to allow a partner to take part in their treatment, while others will allow a partner to be fully involved. It can be helpful if the patient will allow the partner to become knowledgeable about the disease and to receive the support that is needed.

Sterility in men with cystic fibrosis may make relationships particularly difficult as often the man has reduced self esteem. Women with cystic fibrosis may have to choose between pregnancy, which may cause more lung damage and shorten life expectancy, or the loss of the experience of bearing children. These issues may affect relationships between partners and if a couple decides to go ahead with a pregnancy they will need accurate and sensitive counselling, and support throughout the pregnancy. They will need to know what to do if the baby has cystic fibrosis and they need to be fully informed about the implications of prenatal diagnosis so that they can make fully informed decisions on whether to carry an affected child to term.

The impact of progressive decline in health

Many anxieties relate specifically to the progression of the lung disease in cystic fibrosis. Each exacerbation may increase the fear of loss of a previously healthy state and reasonable level of activity. Many adults are concerned with the problems of cross infection and the acquisition of multiresistant organisms such as *Burkholderia cepacia*. No matter how familiar they are with hospital, many adults become anxious about admissions because they associate the need for inpatient treatment with progression of their disease and deterioration, which may force patients to recognise the poor state of their health. Such anxieties associated with deteriorating health may be increased by friends who decline progressively and die early in adulthood.

Some of these problems may be avoided and an independent lifestyle maintained by patients who have their intravenous treatment at home. There are advantages to being at home and continuing with normal work and family life while having treatment, but self treatment is tiring and time consuming. Adults who undertake their own physiotherapy, give antibiotics intravenously and other medications and carry out overnight nasogastric or gastrostomy feeding, may need five to eight hours a day for their treatment alone.[23]

A further issue that causes considerable anxiety is the point where deterioration in health means that consideration for transplantation becomes imperative. This forces patients to face the reality and severity of their condition prior to deciding whether or not they wish to be referred for a transplant with all its associated implications.

Whenever such choices are made patients are likely to experience feelings of loss, health, career and relationships, and general reductions in self esteem and worth. Though medically there may only be one choice, health professionals must recognise that each patient is an individual and an adult, and that they have the right to choose the quality of life that they wish. The role of the health professional is to inform and advise patients so that they remain in control and can make informed decisions about their own lives. Working with and listening to patients, making compromises where necessary, is likely to encourage patient control and adherence rather than professional control and patient non-adherence.[20 21]

Case 3

A young man attended the clinic for the first time in two years. His lung function had reduced from 70% to 20% of the predicted value, he was cyanosed, breathless, and complaining that he was unable to get out of his chair. He was offered admission to hospital for a two week intravenous course of antibiotics, but he refused. His choice was made when he was fully informed of the consequences and he was told that his decision was accepted, but if he changed his mind he was welcome to return to the hospital for immediate admission. A non-critical acceptance of his decision was important because he felt in control. A week later he requested admission where his condition improved dramatically. He felt happy to be in control and generally much better. After this favourable experience he complied better with all forms of treatment.

Death of a cystic fibrosis friend in childhood and adolescence

Though death in childhood is now uncommon it is essential to recognise the needs of children when it occurs. In western society death is a taboo subject which inhibits questions about it, so it is feared by most people and is dealt with by denial by parents and health professionals. Children learn their views of death from their parents and if it is unacceptable to talk about the problem they may suppress their fears and anxieties, which causes even greater problems through misunderstanding.[24] Rinpoche stated that, "Wherever I go in the West, I am struck by the great mental suffering that arises from the fear of dying, whether or not the fear is acknowledged. How reassuring it would be for people if they knew that when they lay dying they would be cared for with loving insight."[25]

Case 4

A 12 year old was admitted to hospital for the first time. She befriended a boy with cystic fibrosis who died two days after she left hospital. At her next clinic visit the nurse specialist asked her mother if she could talk to the girl about the death and the mother refused: "Oh she knows he died but we don't talk about it any more because it will frighten her."

At the clinic three weeks later the girl's mother reported that the girl had stopped doing her physiotherapy and taking her medication for an unknown reason. During an interview with the nurse specialist at this time the girl burst into tears and expressed her fears of dying. Because she thought she was going to die she saw no point in continuing with her treatment. At last she was able to grieve for her friend and to understand her own disease and that she was not going to die when next admitted to hospital. Support was continued by the nurse specialist and social worker, the aim of which was to help her through her grief and to understand the disease. At her next clinic visit, the girl's mother reported that she was accepting all her treatment and working to keep well. The boy's death had caused particular problems because he had complied well with treatment. In the eyes of his friends with cystic fibrosis he should not have died because he took all his treatment. Death came as a considerable shock to many patients and a group of children were given the opportunity to work through their grieving for this patient with the help of the nurse specialist and social worker.

Death and terminal illness

"To cure sometimes, to relieve often, to comfort always."

Anon. (15th Century)

To adult patients coping with death becomes a part of normal life because they repeatedly lose friends. Some will use denial to cope, while others spend time with their friends before they die. It is important that patients themselves choose how they wish to cope with their grief. Some may need support, and encouragement to attend the funeral if it is their wish, while others may need permission not to attend to avoid feelings of guilt; here health professionals may have an important supportive role. They may help patients to grieve for the loss of their friends and to face up to their own mortality, an essential component of the care. Most patients will need or want to talk openly about death at some point, and may often choose a professional who is willing to discuss the subject rather than someone who appears to be afraid of death. It is important for professionals to be sure of their own feelings and beliefs so that they can be open in their discussions with patients.[22]

Anonymous — as cited in Kubler-Ross:[26] "But for me, fear is today and dying is now. You slip in and out of my room, give me medications, check my blood pressure. Is it because I am a student nurse myself, or just a human being that I sense your fright? And your fears enhance mine. Why are you afraid? I am the one who is dying."

Response

Many health care professionals find it difficult to discuss death and dying in any depth with their patients, mainly because they are uncertain about their own thoughts and beliefs.

Books and poems on death, dying and grieving can be very thought provoking and help patients and professionals to discuss their beliefs. The death of another family member or friend can be used to promote discussion. The poem below (Wynn, 1991; unpublished work) was written as a result of considerable

---

The Heavenly World of Cystics

Life with C.F. has much treatment and pain,
physio and needles could drive you insane.

Don't let your life be boring and glum,
But oh what the heck get out and have fun.

Look after your body with all that physio and stuff,
And share your troubles when the going gets tough.

As you get sicker your needs will grow,
Love and support will help you I know.

When the time has come for you to die,
To the heavenly world of Cystics you shall fly.

A friend may come to take your hand,
To lead you across to that other land.

First your old friends you will see,
Amongst the grass and flowers and trees.

Physio, needles and enzymes no more,
For happiness and laughter is all that's in store.

Goodbye my friend I'll see you one day,
When it's my turn to follow your way.

Sarah Wynn

Printed as a Tribute to Andrea who died on the
15th December 1991.

---

experience in caring for young dying people and a heightened self awareness in the author. It is based on the comments and stories told by young people who were approaching death, rather than on any particular religion. Its positive approach to death has helped many chronic respiratory patients to consider their beliefs on the subject of life after death. Literature such as this has been a great benefit to patients and their families.

To the professionals the patient is a child or an adult, but to the parents the person remains their child whatever their age, so before a patient's death parents must be informed about what is happening. They need a chance to discuss their thoughts and feelings about the child's condition and from there they can be guided to understand what is happening. Parents and patients usually prefer information from somebody with whom they are familiar, such as a nurse specialist or a consultant. Although it is not always possible to predict when someone is going to die, an experienced health professional may assess the patient's condition by taking note of clues given by the patient such as a change in the medical condition, a change in personality, or alteration of voice, posture, or increased breathlessness. These clues can create a framework on which to assess the patient's condition and be a basis for discussion about the possibility of death and the need to grieve.

Case 5

A boy aged 18, and his 22 year old brother were both really well with 50%–60% of predicted lung function and required antibiotics intravenously every three to six months. The younger boy's lung function then deteriorated appreciably and he died after a short period. His brother was relatively well, but then started to deteriorate over the following weeks. There were few medical facts to indicate that his condition was changing seriously but it was thought by the nurse specialist that he was likely to die and this view was passed to the parents when they asked. The view was based on observation and in the light of the difficulty of predicting outcome in any individual patient. The mother said that she wished that she had been told before the younger boy had died and could therefore have prepared herself. At this stage the older boy did not wish to discuss his condition and this was respected. He died about a week later having asked about his condition the day before he died.

Response

Health professionals need the ability to listen and to be there for both patients and their families. Some parents choose not to accept that their child is dying and may ask that the patient is not told what is happening. This is difficult as many patients are aware of their condition and use non-verbal communication to convey information to the health professionals. Parents can be told that information will not be given to patients unless it is asked for, but if they do ask, honest and straightforward answers will normally be given.[15] This is an important aspect of the health professional's expertise, and is based on assessment of the patient's knowledge and awareness, which indicates the depth of information which the patient wishes to receive. Use of open ended questions allows patients to take the conversation further. Patients may express their wishes about terminal care, resuscitation, and even their funeral arrangements.

Major fears about dying expressed by patients are those of pain, dyspnoea and general loss of dignity.[16] It is crucial for health professionals to provide honest and sensitive answers to these questions, the aim being to free patients from any distressing symptoms, be they physical, emotional, spiritual or social, and to maintain life at its full potential.[27] Where there is open and honest communication between the professionals and the patient it allows full support and individual discussion sessions for the family as well as the patient.

"Little do they know that the majority of patients are eagerly awaiting the opportunity to talk about everything that is happening and in prospect. If this is denied them the consequent loneliness adds enormously to their emotional isolation and apprehension."[27]

The passage of information from health professionals can be backed up with a variety of non-pharmacological interventions such as relaxation techniques, massage, and aromatherapy. These together with the sensitive use of pharmacological agents, allows the patient and the family to view the period of terminal illness as being one of dignity, and freedom from pain and distress.

Case 6

In the last hour of a girl's life the nurse specialist was involved with the family, and with the proper use of pharmacological agents she was allowed to die peacefully and without distress. The parents were both deaf and dumb but she had a brother and sister who could speak and they were able to convey the girl's physical needs and symptoms which were met by the multidisciplinary team. The parents were taught to use relaxation techniques which enabled them to feel involved, and they quickly learned to calm her breathing when it became erratic and distressing. She died peacefully with all her immediate family present as well as those actively involved in her care. For these parents it was extremely important to give care to their daughter up to the moment at which she died.

Conclusions

"You matter because you are you. You matter to the last moment of your life and we will do all we can not only to help you die peacefully, but to live until you die."[28]

Psychological distress and its effects in cystic fibrosis

Several studies have shown that psychological distress adversely affects patients with chronic physical illness. Appropriate counselling and support during the illness are essential for a better outcome in chronic disease. Keller demonstrated the benefits of a stress management programme in the study on psychological intervention for adults with cystic fibrosis.

In patients with cystic fibrosis it is important to consider psychological care of the physical illness. Nichols suggested that:
- Recovery from illness and mortality may be influenced by psychological distress
- Compliance with treatment regimens and advice may be adversely affected by psychological distress.

The role of the clinical nurse specialist in the management of cystic fibrosis

The aim is to provide continuity and expertise in the care of patients with cystic fibrosis. Unlike the roles of other members of the multidisciplinary team that of nurse specialists may not be clearly defined. They tend to overlap with other members of the team and this enables them to be mediator between patients and professionals. In an attempt to define the role of nurse specialists, the Royal College of Nursing has stated: "The key function of a nurse specialist is to provide direct patient care and to influence other nurses in doing so. The role demands the specialist to be a resource for colleagues and an advocate for the patient."[29]

Analysis of this statement helps to clarify the role and allows the nurse specialist to include education, support, and intervention to ensure the use of expertise and a high standard of nursing care. The introduction of innovative methods of nursing practice which will enhance the patient's quality of life are a further aspect which facilitates implementation of new treatments as rapidly as possible.

Education

This includes:

- The teaching of other health professionals in the hospital and community about cystic fibrosis to improve patient care and to reduce the stress among patients and their families that arises when they encounter inexperienced professionals
- Teaching patients and their families about the disease and its treatment. This is important because knowledgeable patients are more able to make informed choices about their treatment and lifestyles, and this encourages independence, raises self esteem, and gives greater self control over life
- Development of a home intravenous treatment service to enable patients to give their own antibiotics at home safely and effectively; this can increase their independence and ability to maintain a near normal lifestyle[23]
- Education of teachers and employers to promote a better understanding of the disease which will help individual patients to achieve their educational and career ambitions.

These educational goals can be achieved by leading informal seminar groups, giving more formal teaching sessions in groups or teaching individuals as well as making educational publications available.

Support and intervention

Support of patients has a number of related components including social, clinical, emotional, and psychological aspects. Each patient and family are individual in their needs, and therefore support must be carefully tailored to meet those needs and not overstep boundaries perceived by the recipient.

Support should start at diagnosis and continue throughout life, during the terminal phase of life and beyond the death of the patient including bereavement counselling and follow up for family and friends.[30] The nurse specialist may also intervene at many levels other than in routine clinical care with the objective of enhancing the quality of life both during periods of health and illness. Examples include:

- Considering different methods of treatment
- Finding ways of managing the different demands of treatment and personal needs of the individual, which may be as simple as helping them to plan the timing of their treatment in their daily routine
- Providing a practical solution to clinical and social problems
- Acting as an advocate in dealings with other health professionals who may be less aware of the needs and the wishes of the individual patient
- Being with the patient during procedures which cause anxiety or discomfort. This will reassure the patient and allow the other health professional to carry out the procedure without the extra concern of comforting the patient by listening and discussing difficult issues
- To reduce the amount of emotional and psychological distress.

This combination of knowledge, skills, and expertise and close working relationships with patients often means that nurse specialists are the first people to discuss important issues and other socially or emotionally sensitive issues which patients wish to raise.

Case 7

A boy was aware of his deteriorating condition and was particularly anxious about dying before he received his transplant. In discussion with the nurse specialist these issues were aired and it was clear that his greatest fear was death associated with breathlessness and distress. Methods of controlling this distress were explained to him and further discussion took into account his views on resuscitation and ventilation. As a result of this discussion he made the following requests:

- That he should be fully informed about his deterioration
- He should be allowed to choose when he started taking medication to suppress breathlessness and distress
- He did not want to be ventilated or resuscitated
- He wished to die in full knowledge that he was dying and with dignity and comfort.

The nurse specialist was in a position to influence the use of medication and treatments during the terminal phase of this young man's life. The influence brought to bear came from the patient and, importantly, may not have reached the clinical team by any other route, so through this close working relationship with the patient his needs became central to the activity of the multi-disciplinary team.

References

1 Armour S, Andrew ML. *This is our child.* Cooper A, Harpin V, eds. Oxford: Oxford University Press, 1991: 120–31.
2 Dyer J. The role of the cystic fibrosis nurse specialist — a general view. In: David TJ, ed. *The role of the cystic fibrosis nurse specialist.* London: The Medicine Group (Education) Ltd, 1991: 3–10.
3 Whyte D. A family nursing approach to the care of a child with a chronic illness. *Journal of Advanced Nursing.* 1992; 17: 317–27.
4 Black D, Wood D. Family therapy and life threatening illness in children or parents. *Palliative Medicine.* 1989; 3: 113–8.
5 Kubler-Ross E. *On children and death.* New York: MacMillan Publishers, 1983: 60–76.
6 Kleinke C. *Coping with life challenges.* 1990. California Brooks/Gole Publishing Company, 1990: 129–41.
7 Hyland M, Donaldson M. *Psychological care in nursing practice.* Scutari Press, 1989: 157–71.
8 Goodchild M, Dodge JH. *Cystic fibrosis — manual of diagnosis and management.* 2nd ed. London: Bailliere Tindall, 1985: 128–41.
9 Harris A, Super M. *Cystic fibrosis: the facts.* Oxford: Oxford University Press, 1991: 63–9.
10 Patterson J, McCubbin H, Warwick W. The impact of family functioning on health changes in children with cystic fibrosis. *Social Science Medicine* 1990; 31: 159–64.
11 Lavigne JV, Ryan M. Psychological adjustment of siblings of children with chronic illness. *Pediatrics* 1979; 63: 616–26.
12 Thibodeau S. Sibling response to chronic illness: the role of the clinical nurse specialist. *Issues in Comprehensive Pediatric Nursing* 1988; 11: 17–28.
13 Rosenstein BJ. Cystic fibrosis of the pancreas: impact on family functioning. In: *The chronically ill child and his family.* Thomas, Springfield, 1970: 23.
14 Lobato D. *Brothers, sisters and special needs.* London: Paul Brookes Publishing, 1990: 64–74 and 174–85.
15 Lowenfied M. *Play in childhood.* London: MacKeith Press, 1992.
16 Jewett C. *Helping children cope with separation and loss.* London: Batsford Ltd, 1982: 78–105.
17 Pozola KJ, Gerberg AK. Privileged communication — talking with a dying adolescent. *American Journal of Maternal and Child Nursing.* 1990; 15: 16–21.
18 Nichols K. *Psychological care in physical illness.* London: Chapman and Hall, 1984: 38–44.
19 Clinical Standards Advisory Group. *Cystic fibrosis: access to and availability of specialist services.* London: HMSO, 1993: 77.
20 Landau L. Cystic fibrosis: transition from paediatric to adult physician care. *Thorax* 1995; 50: 1031–2.
21 Keller S, Guzman C, Culen L. Psychological intervention for adults with cystic fibrosis. *Patient Education and Counselling* 1985; 7: 263–74.
22 Duncan-Skingle F. The management of cystic fibrosis. *Nursing Standard,* 1991; Feb 13: 32–4.
23 Wynn S. The cystic fibrosis nurse specialist and home intravenous antibiotics

training programme and supervision. In: David TJ, ed. *Role of the cystic fibrosis nurse specialist.* London: The Medicine Group (Education) Ltd, 1991: 17–25.

24 Kubler-Ross E. *One death and dying.* New York: MacMillan Publishers, 1961: 11–33.

25 Rinpoche S. *The Tibetan book of living and dying.* San Francisco: Harper Collins Publications, 1992: R209.

26 Kubler-Ross E, *Death. The final stage of growth* New York: Touchstone, 1986: 25–6.

27 Hanratty JF, Higginson I. *Palliative care in terminal illness,* 2nd ed. Oxford: Radcliffe Medical Press, 1994: 10–34.

28 Spilling R. *Terminal care at home.* Oxford: Medical Oxford Publications, 1986.

29 Royal College of Nursing. *Specialities in nursing: a report of the working party investigating the development of specialities within the nursing profession.* London: Royal College of Nursing, 1988.

30 Cottrell J. The cystic fibrosis nurse specialist in terminal care and bereavement. In: David TJ, ed. *Role of the cystic fibrosis nurse specialist.* London: The Medicine Group (Education) Ltd, 1991: 26–31.

Index